Picturing Personhood

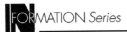IN/FORMATION *Series*

Series Editor
PAUL RABINOW

A list of titles in the series appears at the back of the book

Picturing Personhood

Brain Scans and Biomedical Identity

Joseph Dumit

PRINCETON UNIVERSITY PRESS

PRINCETON AND OXFORD

Copyright © 2004 by Princeton University Press
Published by Princeton University Press, 41 William Street, Princeton,
New Jersey 08540

In the United Kingdom: Princeton University Press, 3 Market Place, Woodstock,
Oxfordshire OX20 1SY

All Rights Reserved

Library of Congress Cataloging-in-Publication Data
Dumit, Joseph.
Picturing personhood: brain scans and biomedical identity/Joseph Dumit.
p. cm. — (In-formation series)
Includes bibliographical references and index.
ISBN 0-691-11397-1 (cloth: alk. paper)
ISBN 0-691-11398-X (pbk.: alk. paper)
1. Brain — Tomography.   2. Brain — Tomography — Social
aspects. I. Title. II. Series.
QP376.6D85 2004
155.2 — dc21
2003042884

British Library Cataloging-in-Publication Data is available

This book has been composed in Sabon

Printed on acid-free paper. ∞

www.pupress.princeton.edu

Printed in the United States of America

10 9 8 7 6 5 4 3 2 1

To my parents, for everything

Contents

CONTENTS

List of Illustrations

Figures

Color Plates
(following page 160)

Acknowledgments

This book has traveled a long way with me and would not have been possible without the wonderful help of my mentors and advisors: Sharon Traweek, Donna Haraway, Gary Lee Downey, Susan Harding, Paul Rabinow, Hayden White, Ramunas Kondratas, Byron Good, Mary-Jo Delvecchio Good, and Michael Fischer. The manuscript has benefited from comments, critiques, and invaluable camaraderie along the way from Marianne de Laet, Warren Sack, Jennifer Gonzales, Ron Eglash, Karen-Sue Taussig, John Hartigan, Angie Rosga, Lorraine Kenney, Chris Kelty, Hannah Landecker, Kim Fortun, Mike Fortun, Anne Beaulieu, Simon Cohn, Nathan Greenslit, Wen-Hua Kuo, Kaushik Sunder Rajan, Regula Burri, Marissa Martin, Amit Prasad, Jake Reimer, Nancy Boyce, Sanjay Basu, and two anonymous reviewers who helped me immensely. Still, all the mistakes and elisions are still mine. Groups, conferences, and seminars have been my intellectual home, and for this project in particular, I want to acknowledge the Galveston Workshop on Scientific Visualization; the School of American Research Seminar on Cyborg Anthropology; the Committee for the Anthropology of Science, Technology, and Computing (CASTAC); George Marcus and the Late Editions groups; and the students of my Brains & Culture classes. Support for this project has come from the Smithsonian National Museum of American History, the National Institute of Mental Health, the National Science Foundation, the Dibner Institute, the Center for the History of Physics. Special thanks to the Dean's Office at the School of Humanities, Arts, and Social Sciences, and the Program in Science, Technology, and Society, at MIT, for supporting the color plates in this book. And the research itself would not be possible without the PET researchers, technicians, graduate students, and journalists, plus many others who talked with me, gave me tours, granted me their time, and tolerated my questions over the years on and off the record. And above all, Sylvia Sensiper has supported, tolerated, motivated, and loved me through this project more than I can ever repay.

Portions of this book are expanded versions of previously published works. My essay, "PET Scanner," originally appeared in *Instruments of Science: An Historical Encyclopedia*, Robert Bud, ed., in the series Garland Encyclopedias in the History of Science, copyright © 1997; it is reprinted here by permission of Routledge, Inc., part of the Taylor & Francis Group. Another essay, "Digital Image of the Category of Person" is taken from *Cyborgs & Citadels: Anthropological Interventions in Emerging Sciences and Technologies*, edited by Gary Lee Downey and Joseph Dumit; it is copyright © 1997 by the School of American Research, Santa Fe, and is reprinted here by permission. I have also incorporated material written by me for two other previously published essays: "Twenty-first-century PET: Looking for mind and morality through the eye of technology," originally published in *Technoscientific Imaginaries: Conversations, Profiles, and Memoirs*, edited by George E. Marcus, and published by the University of Chicago Press in 1995; and from "Objective Brains, Prejudicial Images," published in *Science in Context*, volume 12, no. 1 (1999).

Picturing Personhood

Chapter 1

Introduction

Probably one of the most important initiatives we have ever undertaken is our support for positron emission tomography (PET), an intriguing new research technique. . . . With PET we will be able to examine what happens functionally, in the living human brain, when a person speaks, hears, sees, thinks. The potential payoffs from this technique are enormous.
— Dr. Donald B. Tower, Director of the National Institute for Neurological and Communicative Disorders (from the NIH Record, 1980)

In science, just as in art and in life, only that which is true to culture is true to nature.
— Ludwig Fleck

Sitting in a paneled conference room at the University of California, Los Angeles, with framed brain images on the wall, I am talking with Dr. Michael Phelps, one of the fathers of positron emission tomography (PET) scanning (figure 1.1). As I explain my project on the history and anthropology of PET brain images, he interrupts to turn the question back to me:

PHELPS: What is it? If I am just an ordinary person and I ask you, "What is PET?"

DUMIT: It is a device that is like a CT [computed tomography] scanner but isn't. With PET, you take some molecule or drug that you

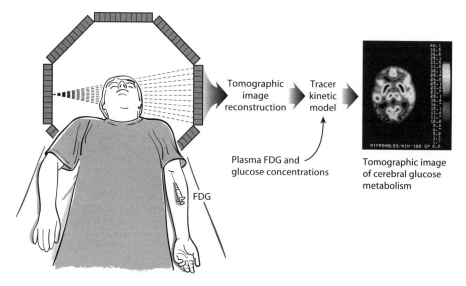

FIGURE 1.1. Principle of positron emission tomography (PET) using example of ^{18}F-fluorodeoxyglucsoe (FDG) to image glucose metabolism in the human brain. (Michael E. Phelps 1991)

want to image—water or glucose, for example. You attach a radioactive isotope to it and inject it into your body, and what you image is where the tagged molecule or drug goes. You image the radioactivity through time; you capture it with a ring of detectors. What you get is an image of a slice and are able to reconstruct where the radioactivity is in one slice that gives a cross-sectional view of where something is through time. You can use it to find out where in the body and with what amounts the molecule is.

PHELPS: You know, another way to approach the explanation is to forget about PET initially and focus on the problem: That is to be able to take a camera and just watch. Inside the body is all this biology that we know is going on. You take food in, you eat it, and it becomes nutrients for your cells.

Your body looks like it is a physical, anatomical substance, but inside there are all kinds of cells that are metabolizing things, or moving around and doing things, signaling to each other. We'd like to be able to watch this action. That is the objective. You know the activity is there, and you'd like to be able to build a camera that can watch it. Well, one way to do that is first to say, "Well, if I was really little, I could go in there, move around, and watch those things." But since you can't go in there, you can send a messenger. So you do that. You say, "Well, I want to look at one portion of this." So you take a molecule that will go and participate in that portion. The molecule will go through that process. You take that molecule and put a source on it that will emit back to you. So you inject it into your bloodstream, and it goes on this journey. It goes throughout your body with the flowing blood, and depending on that molecule, it will go into some organ that uses it. And you have a camera and can sit there now and watch that molecule, watch it go through the blood supply, go into the brain, go into the tissue of the brain, and actually go through the biochemical process. So you have a camera that allows you actually to watch some of that, watch the biology of the body. So that is really the objective. Forget about the particulars of the instruments. I know that inside this being there is a whole bunch of stuff going on, the biological activity of the body, the body's chemistry. It gives me a way to watch that. This is really what PET does. It reveals to us something that we know is going on inside your body, but that we can't get to. And it does it in such a way that does not disturb the biology of the body's chemistry. This molecule is in such trace amounts that it — the body — goes on about its business. The molecule is apparent to us but transparent to the body.

DUMIT: Like an ideal participant observer.

PHELPS: It is an observer that doesn't disturb you. That is, what happens would happen with or without that observer there. If you are an observer at the presidential conference and bother the president, then you distort what would have taken place had you not been there. But this molecule is given in such trace quantities that it makes no disturbance. Whatever happens would have happened whether you were there or not.

PET scans are generated by an incredibly complex, expensive, and deeply interdisciplinary set of techniques and technologies. An experimental PET brain scanner, including a requisite cyclotron to produce radioactive nuclides, costs about $7 million to purchase. A PET research project also needs the expertise of physicists, nuclear chemists, mathematicians, computer scientists, pharmacologists, neurologists. The aim is physiological: to gain information about the patterns of molecular flow in the body at specific places over a specific amount of time. PET scanning is the solution to the problem of how to follow a molecular substance like water, oxygen, sugar, or Prozac and see where in the body it goes, how much goes there, and whether it stays or circulates out of the area. With the use of a cyclotron, radioactive isotopes of one of the four common biological atoms (carbon, nitrogen, oxygen, and fluorine, the latter standing in for hydrogen) are substituted for the original atoms in the molecule of interest. This radiolabeled molecule functions exactly like the normal molecule. As it decays, the radioactivity is captured by the scanner and reconstructed in a map of the flow rate of the molecule. The result is a "picture" of the molecular flow in the body. This description is, of course, very general and overlooks many qualifications, assumptions, and variables in PET. This description is also not neutral. It will take the rest of the book to explain how each description of PET by different PET researchers is part of an ongoing attempt to define the meaning and purpose of PET and PET images, to make claims of invention and contribution, and to give ontological structure to the brain.

As an anthropologist, I have observed and interacted with various facets of this community for over 3 years, and I feel PET to be an incredibly important and increasingly powerful technique for producing images of living human brains. On the basis of my research, I have identified an area of PET signification that I believe is critical in debates over the roles of PET in the world today: *the visual effect of PET brain images*. By attending closely to PET images, I have chosen the most mobile aspect of PET experiments. These images travel easily and are easily made meaningful. Because they are such fluid signifiers, they can serve different agendas and different meanings simultaneously. While representing a single slice of a particular person's brain blood flow over a short period of time, one scan can also represent the blood flow of a *type of human*, be used to demonstrate the *viability of PET* as a neuroscience technique, and demonstrate the *general significance of basic neuroscience research*.

In this book, we will be exclusively discussing PET *brain* images of mind and personhood, which are the most prominent PET images in the media. However, they are only one small part of PET's usefulness. In addition to imaging the brain, PET is used *clinically* to image the heart, to help determine the ability of the heart to withstand a heart-bypass operation. PET is also extremely useful in whole-body and specific organ scanning to detect different cancer types by using a radiolabeled tracer that is attracted to metastatic and not benign tumors (e.g., it has been approved for Medicare and Medicaid coverage to help stage breast cancer).[1] PET is also used in neurosurgery to identify the precise location of epileptic foci. These other uses of PET are not subject to the same kind of critique we will be applying to PET brain-type images. This is because these other uses of PET can be calibrated directly with their referent. The heart, for instance, can be looked at surgically, and in comparison with the PET image one can learn exactly what signals regularly correspond with different tissue states. But in the case of mental activity and brain-types, there is no corresponding calibration.[2] In spite of decades of research into schizophrenia and depression, for example, there are no known biological markers for either one (Andreasen 2001), though with Alzheimer's disease, we may be close. Thus in many cases, though we can say that PET accurately identifies the location of the radiolabeled molecule in the brain, we cannot *verify* that the additional oxygen flow through the frontal cortex is a symptom of schizophrenia.

Popular Brain Images

The brain scans that we encounter in magazines and newspapers, on television, in a doctor's office, or in a scientific journal make claims on us. These colorful images with captions describe brains that are certifiably smart or depressed or obsessed. They describe brains that are clearly doing something, such as reading words, taking a test, or hallucinating. These brain images make claims on us because they portray *kinds* of brains. As people with, obviously, one *or* another kind of brain, we are placed among the categories that the set of images offers. To which category do I belong? What brain type do I have? Or more nervously: Am I normal? Addressing such claims requires an ability to critically analyze how these brain images come to be taken as facts about the world — facts such as the apparent existence and ability to "diagnose" of these human kinds. Behind our reading of these images are further questions of how these images were produced as part of a scientific experiment, and how they came then to be presented in a popular location so that they could be received by readers like us.

As readers, all of the processes of translation of facts, from one location and form of presentation to another, should be imagined when we critically assess a received fact. We should try to become as aware as possible of the *people* who interpret, rephrase, and reframe the facts for us (the *mediators*). We should also critically assess the structural constraints of each *form* of representation — peer review, newsworthiness, doctor presentations to patients (the *media*). In the case of the brain, these processes of fact translation are caught up in a social history that includes how the brain came to be an object of study in the first place, and what factors — conceptually, institutionally, and technically — were part of its emergence as a fact. When did it first become possible to think of the brain as having distinct areas that can break or malfunction? How and when did the brain come to have "circuits"? How did techniques and technological metaphors like telegraphs and electricity make it possible to pose the problem of brain imaging? In turn, what disciplinary and institutional funding mechanisms were available to make the questions posed answerable?[3] Some human kinds that we are starting to take for granted, such as "depressed brains," require attending to broader social and institutional forces in order to understand how it is that we look to the brain for an answer.

An early appearance in the popular media of brain images can be seen in a 1983 article in the fashion magazine *Vogue* (see Plate 1). Entitled "High-Tech Breakthrough in Medicine: New Seeing-Eye Machines . . . Look Inside Your Body, Can Save Your Life," the piece was accompanied by a simple graphic: three similar, oval-like blobs each filled with dissimilar patterns of bright colors (Hixson 1983). Above each shape is a white word in bold font standing out from the black background: NORMAL, SCHIZO, DEPRESSED. The article does not need to be read to be understood. The juxtaposition of words and images brings home quite forcefully that the three colored ovals are brain scans, and that the three brains scanned are different. These images insist that there are at least three *kinds* of brains. Presumably, these brains belong to different people — who are three different *kinds* of *persons* because their brains are not the same. The cultural and visual logics by which these images persuade viewers to equate person with brain, brain with scan, and scan with diagnosis are also the subject of this book.

Facing the brain images in *Vogue*, there appears to be something *intuitively right* about a brain-imaging machine being able to show us the difference between schizophrenic brains, depressed brains, and normal ones. This persuasive force suggests that we ignore the category question of whether three kinds of brains *means* three kinds of people. How could there not be a difference in these three kinds of brains if there are such differences in the three kinds of people, schizophrenics, depressed, and normals? And after seeing the different brain images, how could one not perceive a difference between these three "kinds" of people? The images with their labels are part of the process of reinforcing our assumptions of difference and making them seem obvious and normal. Rationally, we may still remember that this is a category mistake, a substitution of a small set of scan differences for the universal assumption of differences in kind. Thus, the effect of such presentation of images is to produce an identification with the idea that there is a categorical difference between three kinds of humans that corresponds essentially to the three kinds of brains — or *brain-types*. So we see, too, that in our encounters with brain images we come face-to-face with an uncertainty regarding our own normality and "kinds" of humans that we and others are. Alongside the social and institutional components of brain-fact production, we must face this question of how cultural identification and intuition coincide with these representations of reality so that we are persuaded to take them as true.

What does it mean to encounter "facts" like brain images in popular media? How are "received facts" like these used in other contexts and by other people — in courtrooms, in doctors' offices, before Congress? The labels and stories accompanying the image may be far removed from the careful conclusions of the original scientific journal article, and the news story may include comments deemed "indefensible" by the original researchers. Nevertheless, popularization is not a simple one-way process of corrupting by dumbing down a scientific message. In many cases, the researchers will continue to participate with journalists in constructing these stories because there are not many other ways to get the facts out. Publicity in all of its forms, with all of the transformations it conducts on the facts, is how we come to know facts about ourselves (Myers 1990; Nelkin 1987; Prelli 1989). In any case, like scientists, as scientists, we supplement our knowledge with facts, knowing full well that the facts almost always have qualifications. This does not stop us from incorporating these facts, however, and from assuming them and acting on them (Hess 1997; Martin 1994).

Many researchers have pondered how risks, danger, and stereotypes (notions of human kinds) are best explained in cultural terms. Ranking uncertain dangers, acting in the face of contradictory facts, and imagining human kinds and attributes are culturally and historically variable practices (Douglas and Wildavsky 1982; Gilman 1988). Borrowing a term from psychology and semiotics, we can characterize our relationship to culture as *identification*. Rhetorician Kenneth Burke defined identification as the "ways in which we spontaneously, intuitively, even unconsciously persuade ourselves" (Burke 1966, p. 301). As in analyses of ideology, the rightness of facts seems to emerge from our own experience.[4] This notion of self-persuasion helps us keep in mind both the persuasive action of received facts (e.g., from a magazine) and the *form* in which we often (but not always) incorporate them *as facts*.

We might call the acts that concern our brains and our bodies that we derive from received-facts of science and medicine the *objective-self*.[5] The objective-self consists of our taken-for-granted notions, theories, and tendencies regarding human bodies, brains, and kinds considered as objective, referential, extrinsic, and objects of science and medicine. That we "know" we have a brain and that the brain is necessary for our self is one aspect of our objective-self. We can immediately see that each of our objective-selves is, in general, dependent on how we came to know them. Furthermore, objective-selves are not finished but incomplete and in process. With received-facts, we fashion and refashion our objective-selves. Thus it is we come to know certain facts about our body as endangered by poisons like saccharine, our brains as having a "reading circuit," and our fellow human beings as mentally ill or sane or borderline.

Objective-selves always pull at issues of normality, and with brain scans there is a powerful semiotics of what counts as normal. However, normality can be a variety of things. In the history of science and medicine, Georges Canguilhem has described the many different ways in which the "norm" has been crafted. What is normal has been defined as an average in a population, as a typical member, as an ideal type (Canguilhem 1978). In the case of the PET images in *Vogue*, normal does not necessarily mean "healthy"; it means "nonschizophrenic" and "nondepressed." In other words, if you have a test to diagnose an illness, testing positive for the illness usually means you have it, and testing negative usually means you do not; it does not mean that you do not have *any* illness. The qualifier *usually* must be emphasized, because most tests for biological conditions are not 100 percent accurate. They often have both a false-positive rate and a false-negative rate.

Before we can understand what the labels NORMAL, DEPRESSED, and SCHIZO really mean, we have to know more about how they were defined experimentally. Was NORMAL derived by taking a number of healthy individuals and averaging their brain patterns together? If so, does it matter how many individuals were used, or if they were all right-handed, or all male, or all of college age? Likewise, as critical readers or consumers of depression-industry products and services, we would like to know what criteria were used to select individuals as "depressed." In addition to demographic criteria (gender, handedness, etc.), who or what decided that those individual were depressed? Were they depressed for a long time or only recently? Were they actively depressed while they were being scanned? Had they ever taken antidepressant medication? Regarding the image shown, how many of the individuals had brain images that looked like it, and what was the variation in images of depressed people?

Turning from the individual images, we also notice how *together* they argue that there are three different kinds of brains that correspond to the three kinds of brain images. Because the images are so clearly different from each other, they make the additional argument that each brain kind is easily distinguishable, and thus they promise that a PET scan can make a diagnosis—of schizophrenia, depression, and normality, in this case. If we pay close attention to the shape of the images and know that PET images are pictures of "slices" of brains, then we notice that the three images appear to be different slices of the brains, or at least that the three brains are very different in shape and size. In this case we might *expect* that they would, of course, look different. However, we would wonder whether, if we took the same slice in each "kind" of brain, the PET images would look so different. Perhaps each slice has been chosen to emphasize the part of the brain implicated in the condition. How could we tell this? And what slice would be implicated in a "normal brain," then?[6]

All of this is to say that what we come to receive as facts about ourselves are analyzable from a number of perspectives. We might look at the cultural salience of categories like mental illness and gender. We might look at the fundability of different approaches to brain scanning. We might attend to the available metaphors for thinking about brains and people. Though this may seem critical of the science, these perspectives are the same ones from which scientists talk and debate about their work and its dissemination. Scientists continually have to deal with not only the recalcitrance of their instruments and the resistance of the world but also disciplinary constraints, funders and patrons, competitive colleagues, students in training, social mores and values, and lay interpretations.[7] Everyday notions of human kinds help shape what sorts of questions scientists are allowed to ask and what sorts of selection procedures they enact on their subjects. Idioms and metaphors (e.g., flexibility, efficiency, circuitry, and inhibition) are produced in part by cultural uses and travel back into laboratories. It is out of this busy intersection of technical, social, and cultural flows that scientists attempt to stabilize and conduct their experiments, and it is back into the intersection that their results must go.[8]

These flows enable and constrain science at every level of fact conception, experimentation, publication, and dissemination, and reception, but this does not imply that science *is* culture. There is an interplay between popularization processes and scientific inquiry. Science produces facts in spite of and because of these constraints—laboriously, continuously, and creatively. And we fashion our objective-selves with the fruit of this labor in the form of received-facts in our own continuous and often creative manner, no matter how skeptical we are. This way of living with and through scientific facts is our form of life.[9]

In this book, we will investigate brain images as they are presented in a variety of settings, in order to become better-informed science readers and, some of us, better scientists. Much of the disciplines of the history of science and science and technology studies (STS) concentrate on teasing out the difficulties of establishing facts in a particular place and time.[10] These scholars show how creatively and laboriously science is put together. Thus, we will need to investigate the production of images, including specific machines and experiments, in order to understand how, why, and when assumptions are made. We need to understand that there are different kinds of assumptions: (1) necessary assumptions in the absence of settled answers; (2) efficient assumptions in the face of practical and economic constraints; and (3) provisional assumptions because the experiment itself is hypothesis-generating. Using cultural anthropology, in addition to examining how brain images are painstakingly put together, we will also study how they travel from one setting (e.g., a lab) to another (e.g., a magazine) and what meanings they both lose and pick up in the process. Thus we will learn to pay attention to received facts and to how brain images are put to persuasive use in specific contexts.

The lack of ultimate clarifications as to what brain images mean — in abstract or in a particular use — is a consequence of our considering them in use (and potential reuse and thus reinterpretation). Objective-selves, received-facts, and brain-types are thus "*not terms that avoid ambiguity*, but *terms that clearly reveal the strategic spots at which ambiguities necessarily arise*" (Burke 1945, p. xix; emphasis in original). Following Kenneth Burke,

> Instead of considering it our task to dispose of any ambiguity by merely disclosing the fact that it is an ambiguity, we rather consider it our task to study and clarify the *resources* of ambiguity. . . . For in the course of our work, we shall deal with many kinds of transformation — and it is in the areas of ambiguity that transformations take place. (Burke 1945, p. xviii; emphasis in original)

Methods: An Ethnography of Images

How should or can neuroscientists be accountable for their speculations as they travel into print and into courtrooms? How can we account for these speculations, and are these speculations in fact grounded in a shared cultural notion of personhood and human difference? How do we, can we, might we respond to these conclusions regarding ourselves?

Questions of how brain images function in the world and how we are accountable to them have no simple answer. Investigating them requires a combination of cultural anthropology, STS cultural studies, and history. This project began as an interdisciplinary investigation into the process of producing, disseminating, and incorporating PET experiments into our lives. My model was Appadurai and Kopytoff's ethnographic approach to the "social life of things" (Appadurai 1986; Kopytoff 1986). Meaning, from a cultural anthropological perspective, is a lived relation among cultural actors, and to the extent that things such as images and technologies are attributed agency, they, too, participate in cultural exchange. My intention was to trace the various ways in which experiments were designed with assumed categories of people, how they were carried out and interpreted, published in technical and popular literature, and read and incorporated into further experiments, patients' lives, and everyday notions of personhood. Focusing on the images, I set out to study how these scans were desired, laboriously generated, selected, captioned, published, read, interpreted, argued over, referred to, and forgotten.

My primary mode of fieldwork was to "follow" the images around. I started with both images in the media and with image producers. I conducted extensive oral histories with key PET researchers at six different PET labs in the United States. I interviewed many others, including graduate students and postdoctoral scholars, watched experiments being conducted, and observed day-to-day practices. I studied the practices of writing research grants, attended conferences and public lectures, interviewed science editors and other mass-media producers, looked at the use of brain images in courtrooms, and talked to patients and patient-activists about their experiences with scans.[11]

Difficulties with this approach arose immediately. As a complex, multidisciplinary enterprise, PET has multiple, competing identities. PET also has no unitary history, nor even a definition to which a majority agree. In a single article for *Newsweek*, for example, each PET image included was disavowed by other researchers appearing in the same article, as not very meaningful. In addition, PET's controversial use in courtrooms, contested clinical status, and diverse potential in mental-illness communities made it a very fluid object of study. The challenge became to account both for the multiplicity of PET's meanings and practices and for the powerful circulation of the images into different social arenas.

The "field" of an ethnographic study of images must include, then, not only their "biographies" but also what can be called their "virtual community." By using the term *virtual community*, I am borrowing Allecquere Stone's notion of communities that include technologies as vital participants. These communities are dispersed in space, and although each participant is not necessarily connected directly to every other one, they all interact indirectly with each other via technologies of communication (Stone 1992). There are popular theories of person and science that are also the basis of science theorizing. In terms of PET, all those who meaningfully interact with PET images are part of the virtual community. There are laboratories and granting agencies; there are journals and publishing apparatuses; there are machines, brains and people. Finally, there are definitions and demarcations of authority that interweave all of these — science versus (popular) culture, technology versus society, normal versus not normal — demarcations that are shorthand for the ways in which attributions of agencies, functions, and types are

11

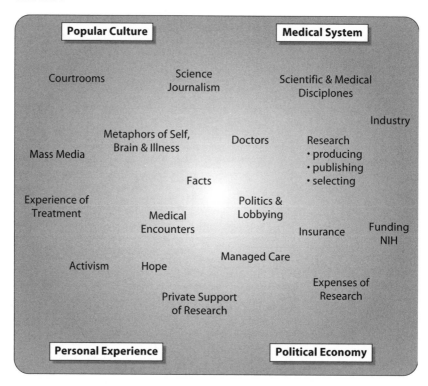

FIGURE 1.2. Virtual community diagram. Heuristic diagram of the "virtual community" of PET brain images. Actors are distributed roughly into four quadrants. The point of this diagram is not to reify the various actors, but to help us keep in mind the wide range of them and their interactions.

distributed, disputed, and constrained. In particular, I am working to locate contests over the true nature of human nature, sites where metaphors are incomplete or excessive and where they are changing. I am interested in the mechanisms of these shifts, their uneven spread, the coexistence of opposing discourses, local existences, and conflicts that involve PET scans.

Because I am interested in the introduction of new facts about biological bodies and brains, I needed to find a way to talk about how the culturally constituted bodily experiences might change (Grosz 1994). In chapter 4 ("Ways of Seeing Brains as Expert Images"), I argue that PET scans are far better suited to show differences and abnormalities than they are to show that someone is normal or that there are no significant differences between groups, and that this inherent preference has powerful consequences when these scans are used in courtrooms. In chapter 5 ("Traveling Images, Popularizing Brains"), I use the concept of objective-self fashioning to look at how facts from science are experienced as objective. In each case, I argue that the consequences of these practices and contests over meaning do, in fact, matter to us. They make important differences in the world.

I also know that these contests are not simply about expert scientists trying to reach consensus over technical issues. Instead, these contests are socially embedded across spheres of activity: mass-media science journalism, mental-illness activism, courtroom admissibility, and widespread readership of published speculations, as well as neuroscientific research. Each of these spheres has its own histories and political economies of the evaluation and dissemination of scientific information. Each of these spheres also has different kinds of stakes in the reproduction of information about the biological makeup of humans.[12]

As an interdisciplinary ethnographer, my interest is in discovering how these different stakes relate to each other, and how these different spheres are connected with and interdependent on each other. My aim is to help evoke these interdependencies and intervene in the ongoing contests over meaning. My position within the virtual community of PET scans is as an anthropologist and historian.[13] I want to evoke the effective and affective *power* that these images, as visual facts, come to have in different arenas of social life, hospitals, mental-illness communities, courtrooms, scientific meetings, laboratories, and in the mass media. And I want to provoke discussion regarding this power. I have been using this position to locate struggles over meaning and power that cross boundaries of expertise and that seem to involve questions of multiple accountability between groups (who do not, themselves, explicitly acknowledge such accountability). Given that the process and outcome of these struggles matters to me personally (as an informed layperson within the virtual community of these scans), one aim of this book is to participate in, and in some cases create, conversations that explain for these multiple accountabilities (Downey and Dumit 1997b).

By respecting both the critical significance of the scientific, technical, and medical expertise and the the implication of public cultural categories in spheres outside of these defined areas of expertise, this book strives to make clear some of the stakes shared — or at least contested — by all participants in PET. Second, I hope to foreground specific current directions of interdisciplinary and intersocial negotiations over the meaning and status of PET images in popular media, mental-illness communities, and courtrooms, in order to raise questions of how these practices might become social problems and begin a discussion on how they might be otherwise.

This work is perhaps best seen as a kind of window into the movements of PET scans in the world: part cultural studies and philosophy (What are PET scans, and how do they function in the world?), part history (How did they arise in these ways?), and part anthropology (How are they meaningful to different communities of people?). As such, it lays the groundwork for more specific cultural projects in the future. In the conclusion, I lay out one such project, looking at the PET functional brain studies of emotions — in particular, sadness and depression.

Two key issues in all big science are money and credit. Grants and publications are the oxygen and glucose, respectively, of research life. They are, of course, both administered through peer review. Alternate forms of funding are both less prestigious and controversial. On the one hand, the PET community is small enough that it is impossible for me to relate specific histories of funding and publication without entering into the local controversies and violating anonymity requests. On the other hand, to tell these histories without the controversies is potentially to perpetuate and/or exacerbate these problems.[14]

Throughout this book are excerpts from interviews I have conducted with PET researchers, from lab leaders to graduate students. Most of these are transcribed quotations from taped interviews that have been edited by both the speaker and myself for readability and accuracy. Others are fieldnotes recorded by me after conversations. In many cases, I do not identify the speaker and have edited out identifying remarks. I have chosen this anonymity to protect those who wished not to be quoted directly and also to evoke a range of positions within the PET community on different issues.

Each of these chapters juxtaposes interview material, semiotic analyses, ethnographic observations, and theoretical reflection. They are written to intervene by engaging. Their tone is exploratory. Like PET neuroscience studies, they are hypothesis-generating, not hypothesis-confirming. Interspersed between most chapters are interludes — conversations between myself and researchers highlighting both the nature of my questioning and the richness of their answers. In general, I prefer long quotations to shorter ones. Long quotations preserve much more of the multiple stakes that researchers constantly negotiate, as well as their explicit awareness of the philosophical, epistemological, and practical aspects of their work.[15]

How This Book Is Organized

CHAPTER 2: METAPHORS, HISTORIES, AND VISIONS OF PET

Chapter 2 provides an overview of the many definitions of PET scanning and, consequently, the many different histories of PET that can be told. On the basis of interviews with three key researchers, PET is variously defined as a pathbreaking technological invention, as a significant direction of research, and as one among many neuroscience tools. Each of these stories of PET conceptualizes the brain in different ways and therefore the kinds of experiments that PET is suited for. With these different basic conceptual notes of what can be studied with PET come different notions of normality, of functions in the brain, and of objective-selves. Each story is also a history and embodies different notions of good science and of scientific progress, as well as the relative centrality of personal contributions. The purpose of chapter 2 is to juxtapose different perspectives while accounting for *how* these views are opposed, in order that a more objective account might be achieved.

CHAPTER 3: PRODUCING BRAIN IMAGES OF MIND

Brain images are produced for a variety of reasons, often contradictory. As with all natural human science, they contain assumptions from a whole apparatus but appear simple and represent types because of the imaging process. In most cases, PET brain-type research is triangulating between (1) groups of subjects selected according to often accurate but imprecise behavioral criteria; (2) the small sampling of the selected populations under study, usually between 4 and 20 people per group; and (3) a "functional" (flow rate) anatomy of the brain that is also imprecise and to some extent unknown at the millimeter level. The resulting PET images, generated at the intersection of these three imprecise referents, are thus paradoxically the most concrete, analytical data available as to whether a behavioral criterion (e.g., a schizophrenia diagnosis) or task (e.g., remembering a number) is reliably handled differently than by the brains of other subjects (e.g., normals) or by the same subjects doing a different task (e.g., resting quietly). The miracle is that we are able to safely and repeatedly get any precise locational data at all about brain functions in living subjects. Historically, no other technique except PET and similar tomographic imagers (functional magnetic resonance imaging [fMRI] and single-photon emission computed tomography [SPECT]) has given quantitative locational information about brain function.

Brain-imaging technologies like PET offer researchers the potential to ask a question about almost any aspect of human nature, human behavior, or human kinds and design an experiment to look for the answer in the brain. Each piece of experimental design, data generation, and data analysis, however, necessarily builds in assumptions about human nature, about how the brain works, and how person and brain are related. No researcher denies this. In fact, they constantly discuss assumptions as obstacles to be overcome and as trade-offs between specificity and generalization. The aim of this chapter is to systematically outline how and where these assumptions are built in so they can be tracked as the images travel.

Properly representing results of these experiments is another balancing act. This time the balance is between the many kinds of audiences who will encounter these complex images: fellow brain-imaging researchers, other neuroscientists, science journalists, and the public. For those publishing brain images, the question is often how to balance the persuasiveness of the visual scans of *simple difference* with the desire for those images to also represent the significance of the experimental data.

This practice of actively constructing images for publication is neither surprising nor new. Similar issues have been observed concerning graphs, tables, digital astronomical images, and physics' images (Jones et al. 1998; Lynch 1993; Lynch and Woolgar 1990). Images are produced and selected for publication to make particular points and to illustrate the argument and other data presented, not to stand alone. They are, in other words, explicitly rhetorical. This is, one could say, the only way one can present images.

Researchers in the same field know this and read each others' images very critically. They go right to the data, methods, qualifications, and statistical results, and they adjust these depending on genre and audience: granting agencies, journals, interdisciplinary forums, and the general public. Observing this practice, I am concerned with the ways in which brain images and their interpretations as referring to brain-types are appropriated and transformed for further use at each stage of image production, selection, and dissemination, scientifically and popularly. Among scientists, this includes looking at how they design their machines and experiments, how they appropriate each other's work across disciplinary lines, and how they cooperate and compete. With each appropriation and subsequent translation, the content of the image, its qualifications and brain-type referent, changes.

CHAPTER 4: WAYS OF SEEING BRAINS AS EXPERT IMAGES

This chapter looks at how American courts have appropriated brain images as useful evidence by incorporating them into the legal category of demonstrative illustration. Surveying the history of the court's use of images, from photographs to X-rays to computed tomography (CT) and PET, we can begin to understand how none of these images were immediately persuasive or understandable. Each kind of image required a "learning to see," by scientists and doctors as well as laypersons.

The persuasiveness and truth status of these learned images before juries is an ongoing concern of the court. Digital brain images are often presented as automatic, computed, and objective illustrations demonstrating insanity and incompetency. PET images thus seem to have a persuasive power that is out of proportion to the data they are presenting. The scans become visual truths, presenting themselves as facts about people and the world such that even their own producers cannot refute them. My suggestion is that the courtroom use of PET images, which most researchers dislike so much, is actually enabled by the way the images are presented by them in journals. Intrascientific communication, in other words, is not a closed world at all but a participant in contests over human nature, rationality, and cause and effect with the rest of society.

We will pay particular attention to how images are recaptioned, decontextualized, and recontextualized, and how they are presented in relation to other images. We do not have to suspect the accuracy of the underlying experiments to recognize that the visual appearance of "graphically" different brain-type images is produced, in part, by a *choice* to visualize the data as *very* different in color. Comparative images are one of the most powerful, persuasive presentations of brain-type data. If nothing else, they visually convey clear-cut graphical difference that *can* be easily *read* in some situations as referring to clear-cut statistical difference or even absolute difference in populations and brain-types. Thus, they *can* help produce, in some situations, the identification of groups as brain-types.

We must emphasize the word *can*, and the form and location of these readings, because we need to be constantly wary of easy assignments of blame for (mis)readings. Scientists take great pains to qualify the meaning of their images (e.g., schizophrenic and normal) and make sure that the conclusions they present do not overstep their data. In this, they are appropriate with the culturally accepted norms of their disciplines. Many of these scientists clearly state in their articles that there is no way, yet, to go from scan to diagnosis, that the correlation is nowhere near being established. Yet most of these same scientists explicitly hate the fact that PET images of schizophrenics can be shown to help persuade juries that a person has schizophrenia. This chapter thus investigates how the visual practices of PET researchers — how they produce, choose, and publish images — enables many of these appropriations that the researchers so abhor.

17

CHAPTER 5: TRAVELING IMAGES, POPULARIZING BRAINS

Chapter 5 builds on all of the preceding chapters to enter into another set of contested meanings involving PET scans. Defining and treating mental illness has a long and troubled history of conflicts, accusations, and accountabilities between biologists, psychotherapists, neurologists, psychiatrists, criminologists, mothers, fathers, families, genes, drugs, communities, and patients. PET scans weigh into these contests as visual evidence of brain differences between those with mental illness and those without it. PET often enters as proof of the biological existence of mental illness in the brain. Chapter 5 follows some of the ways in which this evidence is generated, presented, debated, and incorporated into people's lives. Attending to many issues involved in the political economy of PET research as well as mental-illness diagnosis and treatment, it raises issues regarding concurrent positive and negative effects of PET demonstrations today. In the case of mentally ill patients and their families, the ability of PET to show biological differences promises an understanding of biological origins and the promise of a cure in the long term. In the short term, this "proof" of biological origin both empowers some families to face mental illness as a disease and not a failure of will and has potentially disempowering effects for those who depend on community-based mental-health institutions. Blame and accountability are not easily assigned. But an ethnographic approach to the virtual community of PET scans has the potential to bring different perspectives into conversation, and it can highlight some of the unintended effects of cultural equations and scientific practices.

CHAPTER 6: CONCLUSION

In effect, each of these chapters is a slice through the virtual community of PET scans. Each brings some members of the community into relation with each other and ignores others. Collectively, these chapters aim to evoke the busy intersection between culture in its popular, forensic, and activist manifestations, and neuroscience; to watch its traffic and borrowings; and to draw some lines of accountability between what appears to be gulfs, ultimately, of expertise, of knowledge, and of consequences.[16] I am interested in PET because it is not over — it is still being defined; its purpose is still under debate — because it is part of the rewriting of our received-facts about ourselves as biological, sentient beings.

Interlude 1
Thinking about Reading

Intrigued with brains and the meaning of machines that might be able to record thought processes in the brain (figure 1.3; see Plate 14). Philosopher Ludwig Wittgenstein, in 1936, considered the problem of whether and how we can objectively tell when someone is truly reading. He surmised that perhaps there is no way to tell:

> But isn't that only because of our too slight acquaintance with what goes on in the brain and the nervous system? If we had a more accurate knowledge of these things we should see what connexions were established by the training, and then we should be able to say when we looked into his brain: "Now he has read this word, now the reading connexion has been set up." — And it presumably must be like that — for otherwise how could we be so sure that there was such a connexion? That it is so is presumably a priori — or is it only probable? And how probable is it? Now ask yourself: what do you know about these things? — But if it is *a priori*, that means that it is a form of account which is very convincing to us. (Wittgenstein 1986, §158)

Wittgenstein's exploration of the boundaries of the meaning of *a priori* brings him to culture: We know these things because we have read them in textbooks and heard them from adults whom we trust. "How do we know," he was fond of asking, "that we have a brain, if we have never seen it?"[17] We have, he suggested, a kind of certainty that seems a priori, intuitively self-evident: "Of course, it must be like that." This kind of certainty would be learned (because we are not born knowing about our brains), and yet logical. In order to further explore the limits

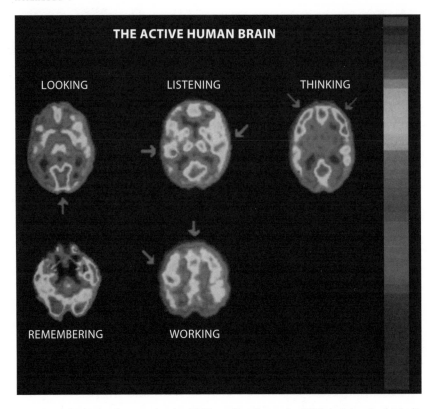

FIGURE 1.3. Active human brain. PET studies from the UCLA School of Medicine showing changes in glucose metabolic function of the brain when healthy volunteers are asked to perform different tasks. (Michael E. Phelps 1991)

of our certainty, consider a variation on Wittgenstein's thought experiment. What if a research team published an article demonstrating that a specific, reliable change in the blood flow of the big toe was correlated with a person's learning to read? This would be greeted skeptically at best, and if it were repeated in person after person, we would not say, "Okay, reading *is* a function of the toe." Instead, we would ask, "Well, what *causes* the blood flow in the toe?" And if we eventually located a correspondence between an area of the brain and the big toe, even if the brain "signal" were weaker and less reliable than the toe "signal," this would then nevertheless confirm to us that reading was in the brain and that the toe flow was a "symptom" of the brain process. But why is it that when we find a reading correspondence in the brain we are satisfied that we are in the right place? Because, suggested Wittgenstein, that is our form of life, our local culture. At certain points (and not others), we no longer ask for an explanation or a test of its truth; explanations come to an end.

Giving grounds, however, justifying the evidence, comes to an end; — but the end is not certain propositions' striking us immediately as true, i.e., it is not a kind of seeing on our part; it is our *acting*, which lies at the bottom of the language game.[18] (Wittgenstein 1991, §204)

Chapter 2
Metaphors, Histories, and Visions of PET

PET Popularity and Phrenology

PET was the first noninvasive technology to permit direct quantitative assessment of regional physiological processes in the brain.[1] In terms of the quest for information about the brain, this was unprecedented and therefore worth investigating.[2] Being complex and ambiguous, PET allowed scientists to make exacting measurements of blood flow, glucose uptake, and dopamine-receptor uptake. Yet fundamental questions remained. What did these measurements actually imply about the purpose and status of the brain and the person?

To put this another way, the human subject can be carefully characterized from the outside — demographics, physical health, genetic history, medical history, nutritional state, mental/emotional state, and behavior. With the development of PET, these characterizations could be correlated with measured information from the brain via a PET scanner. In the process, however, assumptions about two crucial relationships remained: the relation of the measurement to the brain and the relation of the brain to the person.

This is the view of *Newsweek* science editor Sharon Begley:

> Well, I think it does touch a lot of people's imaginations. The idea that you can quote-unquote "see" what a brain is doing during a particular task, that does intrigue people. So apart from what you can learn scientifically, about where glucose is being used in a brain, yes, it does have a sort of man-in-the-street appeal: "Wow, that's a brain

at work, and I can see how it's different when it thinks about an animal and when it thinks about a mathematics problem."

Begley's insight is that with very little prompting, it is possible to conjure up a fascinating possibility, and that this invokes a sublime reaction — "Wow" — a tense combination of imagination and challenging reason. She notes that it is the *idea* of seeing the brain working that intrigues people. Apparently because the idea is already desired, the actual presentation appears as already known, as familiar.

The late William Oldendorf Sr., neuroscientist and innovator in CT scanning, authored a book called *The Quest for an Image of the Brain*, which put into historical perspective the medical-scientific desire for any information about what was going on in the brain, a notoriously refractory organ[3] (Oldendorf 1980). From lesion studies to painful angiography to CT scanning, he traced attempts to draw conclusions from traces of the brain. In one of his last lectures, he even noted the historical shift that accompanied increasing knowledge about the brain. Showing a photograph of Boris Karloff as Frankenstein, he commented that whereas when Mary Shelley wrote the original manuscript in 1818 she devoted only half a page to the construction of the creature, James Whale's *Frankenstein*, which appeared in 1931, devotes half the film to it! He interpreted this as a growing fascination with how we are put together biologically.

A frequent observation made about PET brain imaging is its apparent proximity to phrenology, an eighteenth-century theory of brain localization. A quick survey of popular articles on PET confirms this suspicion. PET experiments are discovering and mapping functional regions corresponding to a moral circuit, reasoning, anxiety, social skills, sexuality, intelligence, learning, language, word generation, color perception, form perception, and various kinds of memory. These are similar to the kinds of faculties mapped by the phrenologists.[4] Interestingly, despite their disdain for the complex speculative conclusions of certain PET articles, PET researchers do not denigrate phrenology but rather celebrate it.

> Phrenology has often been criticized as a pseudoscience because there was absolutely no scientific reason to believe that bumps on the skull were related in any way to the brain tissue that underlay them. But its critics usually overlooked that phrenology was based on an analysis, admittedly crude, of the thought processes and behaviors of our daily lives. (Posner and Raichle 1994, p. 11)

However erroneously, Franz Joseph Gall and his fellow phrenologists were attempting to map the locations of brain functions. Princi-

23

ples from other sciences, such as mechanics and electricity, were applied to medicine. (Andreasen, 1984, p. 148)

The purely fantastic phrenological theories of Gall and Spurzheim stimulated studies that established the concept of the localization of cerebral functions . . . (Premuda 1986)

In essence, these neuroscientists are stating that the phrenological movement raised the right questions, but with the wrong technology. Other psychologists and philosophers, however, appear to be more reticent to describe phrenology positively. Jerry Fodor begins his *Modularity of Mind: An Essay on Faculty Psychology* with the following sentence: "Faculty psychology is getting to be respectable again after hanging around with phrenologists and other dubious types" (Fodor 1983).

In contemporary image culture, the value of PET images is still being debated, partly because fundamental questions about the brain are still unanswered. In particular, the significance and weight to be accorded to individual and group variation has yet to be decided or even properly raised. Some prominent PET researchers include in their presentations pictorial examples of intense variation among normal individuals and plead for caution with regard to generalizations. *Plasticity*, for example, is the idea that the brain is a dynamic functional network that can "re-wire" itself from standard layouts to adapt to injuries and other non-standard obstacles. Plasticity, however, is still a relatively minor phenomenon in both popular and PET theorizing. Instead, circuits are described as hard-wired connections of neurons, clustered together. Historian of brain research, Anne Harrington has suggested that these localization models have survived so well in plasticity, in spite of evidence to the contrary, because they are "easy to visualize and to teach"[5] (Harrington 1992, p. 307).

Overturning the age-old axiom that a picture is worth a thousand words, perhaps these PET images *require* millions of words to be understood! In this way, PET research is actually a quest to characterize and understand what these PET pictures might mean in all sorts of dimensions. They are the starting point, rather than the culmination of this investigation.

History and Definition of PET Scanning

Consider the following three descriptions of PET scanning:

"Positron emission tomography (PET) is a unique medical imaging device that takes pictures of the body's chemical systems in living humans." (Phelps 1991, p. 347)

"Positron emission tomography (PET) is a nuclear medicine imaging modality that consists of the systematic administration to a subject of a radiopharmaceutical labeled with a positron-emitting radionuclides." (Ter-Pogossian 1992, p. 140)

"In fact, I really don't distinguish between PET and SPECT as being two different things. It's just a question of different tracers. Everything is the same except the tracers." (Henry N. Wagner Jr., M.D. 1993, interview).

Starting with just these three notions (and there are more) of PET, the would-be historian is already faced with a dilemma: should he or she consider PET as a specific important technological achievement (a device) as an ongoing process of physiological measurement with positron emitters (an application of a technique) or as part of a set of relatively interchangeable nuclear medicine tools being used to investigate biochemistry?

PET's history is interior to its definitions. Debates going on in the 1990s include the usefulness of collecting data with various radioligands (fluorodeoxyglucose [FDG] vs. oxygen-15 [O-15] vs. labeled neurotransmitter agonists), how to register data (same-subject only, intersubject averaging, and between groups; as well as how to build a normal reference), and then how to analyze this data. These are scientific issues, but I am not sure they can be directly decided. In each case, there is more than the interpretation of data at stake. The opponents in these various debates often have very different conceptions of the nature of data about the mind and brain. They might be called paradigms, after the work of Thomas Kuhn. PET researchers often describe their differences as being from different paradigms. Kuhn's notion of paradigm, however, describes a scientific field in which basic questions regarding the nature of data and relations between basic elements are mostly agreed on by the practitioners (Kuhn 1970). With PET brain studies, this is not the case. PET research often has to simultaneously deal with explaining theories and hypothesis using data and by defining what counts as data. Kuhn described fields of this kind as "pre-paradigm," in which various schools of thought are in creative competition:

Being able to take no common body of belief for granted, each writer . . . felt forced to build his field anew from its foundations. In doing so, his choice of supporting observation and experiment was relatively free, for there was no standard set of methods or of phenomena that every . . . writer felt forced to employ and explain. Under these circumstances, the dialogue of the resulting books was often directed as much to the members of other schools as it was to nature. That pattern is not unfamiliar in a number of creative fields today,

25

nor is it incompatible with significant discovery and invention. (Kuhn 1970, p. 13)

Kuhn's description of researchers explaining their approaches over and over, and directing these explanations, often to actually opposed colleagues, is an apt characterization of PET. PET researchers are constantly inventing new scanner architectures, new analysis techniques, new tracers, and new ways of connecting data to the brain and to behavior.[6] These inventions are not simply incremental improvements but often fundamental changes in the meaning of the results of PET experiments — and they often render results across different scanners and techniques incomparable.[7]

To compile a history of PET, then, one must first come to terms with the definition of PET. My introduction described the trajectory of PET experimental studies but left unexplicated what PET is (where PET ends and other concepts begin), and PET's historical status (its place in the history of science and medicine), and its purpose in the world. At first glance, these seem like moot questions: PET is simply a set of techniques and technologies that permit in vivo functional imaging with positron-emitting radionuclides. But as I shall show, this general definition satisfies no one; it explains neither PET's place in the worlds of science and medicine nor its limits. Rather, there are many concurrent, competing definitions of PET, each with not only ontological and teleological but moral and practical consequences as well.

Primarily using the voices and writings of researchers, this chapter investigates each of these questions. My aim is to lay the groundwork for an informed history of PET. In Kantian terms, I am sketching out the conditions for the possibility of a history of PET. I do this by asking the following questions: What is at stake in these contests over PET? How do they set the conditions of possibility for thinking and doing interdisciplinary science work? And how do these contests impact the kinds of questions we ask of ourselves in order to understand ourselves?

In the rest of this chapter, I present four different stories of PET scanning that illustrate fundamentally different notions of the meaning of PET and of its history. The first is a short overview of the history and definition of the PET scanner that I wrote for the *Encyclopedia for the History of Scientific Instruments*. In technical and dense language, it attempts to capture the complexity of PET scanning within its multidisciplinary development. This is followed by three accounts based on life-history interviews with key scientist-participants as well as their published accounts of PET, its development, and its definition and purpose (Thompson 1988). The three interview subjects presented here are Michel M. Ter-Pogossian, Michael Phelps, and Henry N. Wagner Jr.

They were chosen in part for their clear roles in the development of PET and for their very different disciplinary orientations. They make it clear that the act of telling a history is a way of defining what counts as an event and what does not. Reading and listening to these histories, one must appreciate the role that metaphors and narrative frames play in defining projects one way rather than another. These histories are thus ethnohistories, perspective-dependent accounts told within a contested field.

PET Scanner: A History in One Thousand Words*

PET is an acronym for *positron emission tomography*, a set of techniques and technologies for obtaining tomographic images (slices) of molecular biological activity in living beings. In contrast to CT scanning, which provides structural information about bodies (e.g., bone density), PET provides functional, time-dependent images of the rate of flow of specific molecules through a particular area of the body. PET thus provides a solution to the problem of how to obtain useful information about biochemical processes taking place in relatively inaccessible sections of living organisms (e.g., the heart and brain). The information that PET presents is both quantitative and visual, demanding careful measurement and complex physiological modeling in order to be interpreted.

PET is currently used in a variety of clinical studies, including heart tissue viability, epilepsy focal localization, bone and breast cancer detection, and head trauma diagnosis. It has also been used in psychophysiological studies — correlating oxygen blood flow in specific regions of the brain with motor movement, visual attention, and cognitive tasks, as well as more complex cognitive skills. In psychiatry, Seymour Kety, David Ingvar, Monte Buchsbaum, and Jonathan Brodie each led teams that conducted extensive studies of schizophrenia. Other mental disorders have also been imaged. These have stimulated speculation on possible biological or molecular explanations of these disorders, but diagnostic ability still eludes investigators.

PET is located at the intersection of a number of disciplines and technical paradigms. Though they are numerous, it is perhaps better to gesture toward the complexity than exclude, outright, vital participants. One strand fundamental to functional imaging is the biological tracer technique for which Georg von Hevesy was awarded the Nobel

* This material is adapted from an essay entitled "PET Scanner," by Joseph Dumit, which originally appeared in *Instruments of Science: An Historical Encyclopedia*, Robert Bud, ed., in the Garland Encyclopedias in the History of Science, copyright © 1997; it is reprinted here by permission of Routledge, Inc., part of the Taylor & Francis Group.

27

prize in 1944. Hevesy detailed the means whereby a radioactive isotope of a molecule could be used in place of that molecule because it is chemically *indistinguishable*, yet its radioactivity can be tracked. This technique was used in medical physics and later in nuclear medicine, first to follow molecules and later to image their distribution. Unlike X rays, which are produced externally in tubes and transmitted through organisms in order to reveal their structure, these radioactive tracers emit their rays from within. Early detection of the pathways of these tracers was with Geiger-Mueller (gas discharge) tubes, and later through scintillation counters — crystals that react to radiation by discharging photons or light that is then converted to electricity where it is measured. A significant advantage in data gathering was the rectilinear scanner by Benedict Cassen in 1949, which rapidly and precisely took measurements over a bodily area in a zigzag fashion. Around the same time, Harold O. Anger introduced a scintillation camera consisting of multiple scintillation tubes simultaneously collecting data. Both of these devices produced images on film consisting of spots, either darker or lighter relative to the quantity of emission. Improvements on Anger's gamma camera were followed by devices using more scintillation counters, arranged and collimated (filtered) to provide better three-dimensional specificity.

Another strand of innovation concerned developing better and more specific tracers. Chemists, nuclear chemists, and physiologists were seeking to follow specific biological processes and needed to tag certain molecules (chemicals such as water or pharmaceuticals) either with radioactive isotopes of constituent atoms or with close analogs of those atoms. One class of isotopes is known as positron emitters because its constituents decay radioactively into positrons that travel a few millimeters, collide with an electron, and result in a mutual annihilation, producing two 511-KeV (kiloelectron volt) gamma rays that travel almost exactly 180 degrees away from each other. These positron emitters (carbon-11 [C-11], nitrogen-13, [N-13], oxygen-15, and fluorine-18 [F-18]) were initially explored around 1939, by Martin Kamen and Samuel Ruben, who then discovered carbon-14 (not a positron emitter) and stopped investigating the others. The positron emitters were difficult to work with for a number of reasons. For instance, they have very short half-lives ($C - 11 = 20$ minutes; $O - 15 = 2$ minutes; $F - 18 = 2$ hours) and they must be produced with the aid of a cyclotron, and bound or tagged onto molecules before being introduced into the organism.

The postwar policy of the Atomic Energy Commission (AEC) promoting the peaceful use of radioactivity was the context for exploring positron emitters within medical research. In 1951, Frank R. Wrenn and colleagues proposed that the two gamma rays produced could be detected simultaneously to provide very accurate location of the tracer—for instance, to localize brain tumors. In 1953, Gordon L. Brownell and William H. Sweet at Massachusetts General Hospital built a positron scanner to do just that. In the early 1970s, James S. Robertson at Brookhaven National Laboratory built the first positron camera with detectors arranged in a ring. In the same year David Kuhl and R. O. Edwards at the University of Pennsylvania developed a tomographic imaging device for single-photon (gamma-ray) emission. These set the stage for fully developed PET scanning.

Physiologically, work with positron emitters was carried out by Michel M. Ter-Pogossian and colleagues at Washington University in St. Louis in the 1950s and 1960s, using O-15 gas (O_2) for respiratory, brain, and cancer studies. These lead to the installation of a cyclotron in the George Washington University Medical Center in the mid-1960s, with support from both the AEC and the National Institute of Health (NIH). In the late 1970s, Louis Sokoloff, working at the NIH and building on the work of Seymour Kety, contributed the autoradiographic technique using deoxyglucose as a tracer, which allowed them postmortem to "see" oxygen flow in the brain precisely.

The precipitating event for the PET scanner was the announcement of the CT scanner by EMI, which demonstrated the feasibility of solving the computational problem of how to filter tomographic data using a computer. With this inspiration, Michael E. Phelps and Edward J. Hoffman, along with Jerome R. Cox, Donald L. Snyder, and Nizar A. Mullani, developed the first practical PET scanners, the PETT series (for Positron Emission Transaxial Tomograph), under the leadership of Ter-Pogossian. These devices consisted of a hexagon of scintillation detectors that were electronically linked so that they sent a positive signal only when two opposite ones detected a gamma ray at the same time. When this happened, it could be assumed that there was a positron-emitting molecule somewhere along the line between the two detectors. These signals were stored in a computer and then processed mathematically using first an iterative algorithm and later Fourier transforms to reconstruct a two-dimensional (tomographic) slice of the radioactivity. Coincidence detection thus substituted electronic collimation for the physical lead-shield collimators used in gamma cameras. This improvement provided significantly more sensitivity and accuracy. Critical improvements in this technology included the practical discovery, by Z. H. Cho, of bismuth germanate (BGO) crystals for better detector resolution and the use of a stationary ring of detectors rather than a moving hexagon, which provided for easier engineering.

To be used medically, however, this data had to be further processed in terms of the complex relationships between the molecular circulation in the body, radioactive decay, and the process to be studied (e.g., the relationship between oxygen concentration in blood, bloodflow in specific areas of the brain, and cognitive processes). This parametric calculation/estimation is known as tracer-kinetics. The resultant image is called *functional* because it purports to show the rate of flow of a molecule, its concentration through time in a set of regions.

The usefulness of PET depended equally on radiopharmaceutical constraints and on technological ones. Much research with PET concentrated on ligand work, developing ways to rapidly tag complex molecules, such as pharmaceuticals, to show how and where they are used in the body, especially where they are absorbed in the brain. A significant advance came in 1979, when Joanna S. Fowler, Alfred P. Wolf, and David E. Kuhl synthesized and used 18-FDG, an analog of glucose, to approximate glucose consumption in the brain. This has become the most-used radiopharmaceutical in PET. Another significant advance was the demonstration of the ability to image human dopamine receptors, carried out by Henry N. Wagner Jr. and Michael Kuhar at Johns Hopkins University in 1983.

Following the development of the PETT devices, commercial PET scanners were developed, first by EG&G Ortec (which became CTI). In 1979, the NIH funded seven PET centers under a program grant, initiating PET as a subfield. In spite of this boost, PET did not enter clinical medicine in the explosive way that CT did. Rather, because PET required a tremendous interdisciplinary and financial infrastructure, including an on-site cyclotron, and because its data was not immediately applicable for clinical solutions, the procedure became first a scientific and medical-experimental technique. Nonetheless, by 1983, the number of PET centers in the world exceeded forty. The mid- to late 1980s found established medical device providers Siemens and General Electric, taking over the marketing of the PET devices of the two largest PET providers, CTI and Scanditronix, respectively.

PET, along with SPECT, is located in an interdisciplinary space contested by radiology and nuclear medicine. These new imaging devices have also facilitated new disciplinary formations, such as medical imaging and molecular pharmacology — the latter understood as the tracer-imaging counterpart of molecular biology.

In popular culture, PET's ability to provide pictures of the brain in action, as a person performs a cognitive task, and to image different kinds of brains (diseased, disturbed, disabled) have captivated the imaginations of science journalists and Hollywood screenwriters.

Courtrooms have recently been faced with the issue of PET's admissibility as scientific evidence in head trauma and insanity cases, as well as the vexing question of the possibly prejudicial status of PET images for juries.

In the early 1990s, efforts were under way to make PET a "clinical" technique, which means having insurers, especially the Health Care Financing Administration (which administers Medicare and Medicaid) cover the cost of procedures done with PET. Although there was progress in this regard, the issue of coverage depends on cost as well as on clinical efficacy: Will enough hospitals be able to afford PET so that everyone has access to approved procedures? The cost of a PET scanner is around U.S. $2 million dollars, the same as for a cyclotron. Yearly maintenance and personnel costs (a cyclotron crew, chemistry and PET crew) can cost $300,000 to $700,000 per year. Some of this cost might be reduced with the introduction of regional cyclotrons delivering radioisotopes to groups of nearby hospitals. Additional challenges are being worked out at the regulatory level, with the U.S. Food and Drug Administration (FDA) trying to decide the status of radiolabeled molecules. Finally, there are other techniques of imaging bodily and brain functions (e.g., SPECT and fMRI), which overlap some of PET's strengths.[8]

Toward an Ethnohistory of PET

The above history represents my attempt to abstract (1) a concept of PET as a scientific instrument, (2) the involvement of a number of people with its development, and (3) the current status of PET and its role in social issues. According to the editors of the *Encyclopedia for the History of Scientific Instruments*, I had to write the history using less than nine thousand words. The article appears as an objective, historical narrative, in the third person, past tense.

However, as I conducted my research, I found that the more people I talked with, the more people I should have talked with. It quickly became clear that to write a history of PET was to take sides in what PET really is and should be. At first it appeared as if the matter could be solved simply by deciding who was right, who really invented PET. But instead of a mystery, I found multiple stories and heteroglossia. The anthropologist in me soon realized that I was actually dealing with competing ethnohistories. Ethnohistory is itself a contested branch of anthropology and history. Gewertz described it as "fundamentally tak[ing] into account the people's own sense of how events are constituted, and their ways of culturally constructing the past"[9] (Gewertz and

31

Schieffelin 1985). In fact, scientists are quite aware of their histories as strategic modes of storytelling:

DUMIT: That is why I have to talk with a number of people.

PHELPS: And it makes sense. This is not a unique situation, this is one more of science. You know we were all in Cologne, Germany, last year, where all of us were on the program. And part of the program was "History of PET." There is an older group, you know, Al Wolf, Mike [Ter-Pogossian], people in the generation before me. They got up and went through things. Ter-Pogossian took it from — and you know this was his own choice, he chose where to start and cut — he took it from his work in introducing the cyclotron into medicine, developing the initial positron-labeled compound studies. He did not show that he developed PET. Now everybody there knows he didn't dare do that. But he contributed to PET. Without these things that came before me — I mean, I came into a lab that he developed; he developed a lot of this — had he not done that, I would not have gone on to do my part.

DUMIT: That is the challenge of writing history — trying to figure out not only how to be fair but [also] figuring out where to cut, what kinds of stories of causation and seeds and so on.

PHELPS: You know, science tends to be an evolutionary concept. It depends on one's religious beliefs. I mean, there is supposedly only one creation. Truly from nothing before to now, but science doesn't typically do that. That is a religious experience if it is really truly an absolute creation. You know there are things that other people did before you. And there are certain benefits that come to you from the influence of people on what you are doing. Then there are certain portions where you put it in, and that's your contribution. But when laid out in the evolution of science, you know you are just pieces in this.

To investigate the variability of this history, I chose three key researchers who each have their own ethnohistory of PET and who have all been described as fathers of the field, keeping in mind that there are many more who might also be chosen.[10]

Michael E. Phelps

PET was originally developed by Dr. Michael E. Phelps, Jennifer Jones Simon Professor, chief of the division of nuclear medicine and biophysics and director of the Crump Institute; and by Dr. Edward Hoffman, professor of radiological sciences. (Harris 1990, p. 16)[11]

Michel M. Ter-Pogossian

The first useable positron emission tomography (PET) instrument for human studies was developed in the early 1970s by a team of researchers led by Michel M. Ter-Pogossian, Ph.D., at Washington University's Mallinckrodt Institute of Radiology in St. Louis. (Welch and Gold 1989, p. 2)

Michel M. Ter-Pogossian, Ph.D., professor of radiation sciences, is affectionately known as "the father of PET." (Welch and Gold 1989, pp. 6–7)

Henry N. Wagner Jr.

Although the field's forefathers, Glenn Seaborg, Benedict Cassen, and Emilio Segre, have passed away, many of the founders of nuclear medicine as a scientific and medical specialty remain vital and involved. No one better defines this founding role than Henry N. Wagner, Jr., M.D., whose career nearly spans nuclear medicine's "second 50 years," as he termed the period in a 1996 account of the field. Present at the origins of nuclear medicine as a defined sector of medicine, Wagner has sustained the momentum of discovery that began in the 1950s and 1960s. He has promoted nuclear medicine at key U.S. teaching and research centers around the world, including his own Johns Hopkins School of Medicine, where he continues to serve as a professor of environmental health sciences. ("Biography of Dr. Wagner"[12])

The first two, Phelps and Ter-Pogossian, were both at Washington University in the early 1970s, and both have been called inventors of PET; both received awards to that effect by the same societies, and both headed PET programs.[13] But Phelps was once a postdoctoral candidate working for Ter-Pogossian during the time that the first PETT scanners were developed. Without exception, every researcher alluded to the competitiveness of the field and mentioned that at times it had been quite destructive.

> RESEARCHER: I'm sure you are getting a sense, because you are doing it historically and talking to a number of people, of the intense competition.
> DUMIT: Some of it.
> RESEARCHER: It is like with Watson and Crick, who for all intents and purposes left out the contribution of Rosalind Franklin. Listening to the story of Ter-Pogossian and Phelps is very reminiscent. I've heard them give their history of PET talks, and well—are we talking about the same discovery?!
> DUMIT: Right. I've learned enough about the situation that when they talk, I can hear differences, some of the silences, the reluctance to talk about the other person.
> RESEARCHER: From what I understand it was a difficult time.

The carefully crafted sentence in my thousand-word history dealing with this set of events reads:

With this inspiration, Michael E. Phelps and Edward J. Hoffman, along with Jerome R. Cox, Donald L. Snyder, and Nizar A. Mullani, developed the first practical PET scanners, the PETT series (for Positron Emission Transaxial Tomograph), under the leadership of Ter-Pogossian.

What follows is a set of accounts of PET by Phelps, Ter-Pogossian, and Wagner drawn from oral histories, published interviews, and scientific articles (Latour 1987; Shapin and Schaffer 1985). My aim here is to unpack PET as a scientific project from the points of view of many of its practitioners. I will abstract their visions to use them as extreme images to represent some of the diversity of definitions and consequences of PET. These are all stories of PET, but they are also weighty stories. They matter for what PET is, for how it is practiced, and for what kinds of meanings are produced through it. Rather than telling a story of scientific development as an agonistic struggle between scientists who compete by amassing more powerful allies than anyone else, one of my purposes is exploring the contested narratives of history and science put forward by these scientists.[14] I am interested in the insinuation of PET into the fabric of practicing neuroscience and psychiatry, as well as into the practices of objective self-fashioning. Finally, these distinctions will aid in understanding some of the debates over clinical and forensic usefulness that are taken up in the rest of the book.

MICHAEL E. PHELPS, PH.D.
PET AS TECHNOLOGICAL BREAKTHROUGH,
SCIENCE AS RATIONAL REVOLUTION

For Phelps (in abstraction), PET is the imaging technology that broke the "4-minute mile" in nuclear medicine:

> Within his remarkable capacity to summarize the entire content of the annual meeting of the Society of Nuclear Medicine, Dr. Henry Wagner, at the 1980 meeting, described the "Banister phenomenon." Before Banister ran the 4-minute mile, everyone said it couldn't be done. However, once Banister did it, the recognition that it was possible allowed others to not only equal but exceed Banister's accomplishment. Thus, once a task is recognized to be within our capabilities and is worthy of the effort, it can become a matter of practice. The development of x-ray CT showed that an enormous mathematical problem and a precise physical measurement could be achieved in both a fundamental and practical manner. With the recognition that it could be done and with the importance of the information it pro-

vided, x-ray CT has become commonplace. It would now appear that we are beginning to recognize the Banister phenomenon in PT [physiologic tomography, Phelps's acronym for PET]. The technique of PT is unquestionably more difficult than x-ray CT, but the type of functional information it can potentially provide has never been more accessible before in studies of man. (Phelps 1981, pp. 47–48)

Drawing on the example of a breakthrough demonstration, Banister's running of a 4-minute mile, Phelps likens scientific progress to a series of such demonstrations. Without them, science slows to a crawl; with them, it leaps ahead. The primary agents of scientific progress in Phelps's narrative are methods of gathering information, specifically for measuring biochemical activity in humans. He begins his introduction to PET (called emission computed tomography, or ECT) in the 1981 *Seminars in Nuclear Medicine* with a characterization of nuclear medicine as a discipline of information that is being threatened by new information technologies from another discipline, radiology.

> Nuclear medicine originated from the efforts of scientists developing methods that used the principles of tracer kinetics to study physiologic processes with compounds labeled with radioactive isotopes. Since that time nuclear medicine has grown into a successful diagnostic discipline through advancements in radiopharmaceuticals, instrumentation, understanding of human physiology and disease processes, and the unique type of information provided by this specialty.
>
> However, the recent development of competitive diagnostic modalities such as x-ray CT, ultrasound, and other techniques such as nuclear magnetic resonance (NMR), along with the desire for self-improvement, is providing the incentive to look for new ways to employ the unique capabilities of nuclear medicine. This is bringing together the multidisciplinary components of nuclear medicine to employ the fundamental principles of their disciplines to new technologies. (Phelps 1981, p. 32)

The polemical motivating agents in this passage are technologies from other disciplines that have encroached on nuclear medicine's diagnostic turf. Nuclear medicine's response has been to develop new technologies of its own. This saving technology, for Phelps, is PET, which draws on CT, tracer kinetics, and new positron-labeled tracers. Phelps continues by highlighting why PET technology is so important: It provides a new kind of information.

> Where the importance of the tomographic delineation of overlapping structures is most often highlighted; it is the fact that the technique allows a type of measurement that was not possible before that

is probably its most important facility, that is, the capability to measure the local tissue radioactivity concentration. . . . Thus, ECT provides a noninvasive approach to apply the principles of tracer kinetics
to man for the assessment of local biochemical and physiologic function if appropriate labeled compounds and tracer kinetic models are
employed. This approach will be referred to as physiologic tomography. If this goal can be realistically achieved, nuclear medicine will
provide a method of investigation in man that has, for the most part,
eluded other modalities. (Phelps 1981, p. 33)

PET, for Phelps, is thus a unique technology that provides information desired but unattainable by other means. The operative metaphor
here is one of an obligatory point of passage (Latour 1987). Before
anyone could advance beyond the barrier of the 4-minute mile, someone had to show that it really could be done. From then on, all scientists can and must pass through this point in order to pursue research
along these lines. The work of tinkering, striving, making something
actually work becomes the true gift of a scientist to his or her field.

In the following passage, taken from an interview with Phelps, he
describes how learning about the brain is dependent on the technology
available. From this observation, he is able to characterize the nature of
the progress of science:

> The activation studies—brain mapping—are a program that says
> we would like to just understand the macroscopic way . . . the brain
> is organized and how it works. So both PET and MRI are developing
> and pursuing ways to just map out how the brain does what you
> know it does. In fact, the first brain-mapping studies were that [point-
> ing to display on the wall] publication in *Science*. That was in 1984
> or '83, I think. In fact, when the cover of *Science* had the MRI on it,
> that was 10 years to the day. And that is a science study where it says,
> "We'd like just to know how the brain is organized and functions."
> Over on the other side is the issue dealing with the merger of biology
> and imaging. You use the techniques you have to learn about things
> and then go develop new techniques to learn things that you have
> never known before.
>
> The greatest turning points in science come by the development of
> a new instrument to allow one to look at things that you have never
> seen before, or a new theory that says, "I have collected all the under-
> standing and knowledge of this and I have built a way to make it
> make sense. It is within this framework, now, that you can collect
> data and interpret it and understand what it means. So, theories and
> instruments. Of course, around all of that are good scientists that
> work every single day to use them to understand. And they aren't
> focused on the instrument but on its use.

Instruments effect great changes in science because they change the kind and amount of information available, and theories effect changes by providing paradigms within which to understand the data. The actual understandings are up to the scientists who apply these fundamental technologies and theories to the world. For Phelps, then, the history of PET involves three stages: the techniques and technologies developed before PET, the actual making PET work (showing what can be done), and then the development of uses for PET. I asked him about the place of PET in history:

> DUMIT: I am trying to envision different ways of telling the development of PET, in terms of different disciplines, different uses of it.
>
> PHELPS: Yes. Its development: there is a basic technology developed, and then there is the development of its use in various problems. You know, before PET imaging really came about, there was a need for accelerators, cyclotrons, to come into medicine, and for the use of positron-labeled compounds to be of some value. Ter-Pogossian contributed a great deal to that. When it comes to the PET scanner and imaging, that begins with mine and Ed [Hoffman]'s efforts to do that. And there were some predecessors to just imaging with positrons: Gordon Brownell and a number of people. But when it comes to PET, that we did.
>
> And then you look at the brain, and you say, "What are the major events in the use of PET?" One of them was the development of the deoxyglucose technique. There you come to the fact that Lou Sokoloff, Brookhaven National Lab and University of Pennsylvania, came into it. Joanna Fowler and Alfred Wolf found a way to make a PET form of deoxyglucose. That was a major event. There is no compound used as often in PET as fluorodeoxyglucose.

Phelps was one of the people to stay up nights pondering, tinkering, and constructing a device that would make computed tomographic measurements of positron tracers. Along with Edward Hoffman, Phelps showed that what had been envisioned could really be done.[15] He broke the 4-minute mile. Phelps's story highlights the technologies and techniques that enabled PET to be built and then the uses to which PET was put.

In the following passage, Phelps reveals a *difference* between breaking the 4-minute mile and building a new scientific instrument. While the run is public and clearly acclaimed, the device is private and must be proven over and over before skeptical audiences:

> PHELPS: Quite frankly, in those early days we had done things driven by our imagination and our ideas. We had worked day and night. In fact [pointing at a photograph on the wall], that first scan with

37

PETT III we took at five in the morning. It was supposed to be a circle. We were excited about it, but it didn't turn out to be a circle.

DUMIT: It was a phantom.

PHELPS: Yes, it was a phantom — we knew the right answer; we didn't quite get it. But it was the first image we got on the PETT III. Then I went out into the world to preach this idea. With a great deal of belief and confidence in it but with very little data. And I was met with a world not . . . ready for this.

DUMIT: Where did you go?

PHELPS: Oh, I went to a great many scientific meetings. I gave the first scientific paper on PET that was ever given, ironically, here in San Diego. I mean nobody had ever heard of PET before, at that time.

You know, everybody talks about how great creativity and originality is, but the dark side of creativity is destruction. If you create something new, you are going to displace or replace something old. You begin with the majority of people in the old and a minority of people in the new, and they don't like it. What comes then is the struggle that is a necessary part of any original development. You have to struggle [. . .] to give birth, to nurture, mature, and bring forward your ideas, realizing that a majority of people are opposed.

The historical turning point or scientific catalyst will be the new source of information and the device that provides it. The challenge to its inventor is to gain the recognition for it from peers who are not prepared to change their perceptions or their stakes to accept this new information. In fact, Phelps describes most of science in this vein of difficult revolution:

PHELPS: Although we did the first brain mapping, we didn't pursue it that much. So there is an initial thing that we did with PET, to show that it could be done; but Mark Raichle [at Washington University] really pursued brain mapping devotedly.

And then you look at the ligands to identify neurotransmitter receptor systems in the brain. When we all started with that, everybody said it is not possible, that the concentrations of the receptors are way too low.

DUMIT: Not possible in terms of the NIH saying there is no funding for this?

PHELPS: The scientists were saying it is not going to happen, and you are not going to get any money to do it.

But even though receptor concentrations are extremely low, one of the values of PET is that we can assay very, very low concentrations. We have that label put on a very sensitive signaling approach. We don't disturb the system, and we can see very small numbers. But even we—all of us in PET—had a question about whether we would be able to do it. And there Johns Hopkins [under Henry Wagner] played a major role. They really built the approaches and demonstrated for people that it could be done. Hopkins did that, a really powerful thing.

The technology of PET is difficult to demonstrate, and it is equally difficult to demonstrate each new technique that makes use of it. For Phelps, proof of the technological achievement of PET and of the techniques that followed it lies in the fact that people have taken them up and pursued them.

Proving a new technique to an unreceptive audience is not easy, however. Often it is the source of controversy. Controversies have long been used in STS to gain insights into the practice and maintenance of science and discovery (Nelkin 1979). Among scientists, stories of controversies have a similar function, to pass on insights about the real practice of science.

The controversy narrated below by Phelps concerned the meaning of deoxyglucose activity in the brain, specifically whether or not it was a reliable, precise, and accurate indicator of glucose consumption.[16] It appears to have been resolved in Sokoloff's favor,[17] but continues to be raised as an example of PET's and/or FDG's possible unreliability.[18]

You know, when Lou Sokoloff developed the deoxyglucose autoradiography technique for animals, it was a phenomenal breakthrough. But there were many people that attacked the method—and attacked Lou—with lots of different agendas. He went through a hell of a struggle. When he went into the National Academy of Science—you have to give a talk on your work—and one of the laureates of physics got up and said that he didn't know much about deoxyglucose, but he was curious whether the technique had been used to teach us about behavior and its relationship to the brain. And Lou paused for a minute, and he said, "Well, I'm not sure how much the deoxyglucose technique taught us about behavior, but I'll tell you that *developing* it has certainly taught me a lot about behavior!" Because the more and more successful it became, and the more popular, the more there were people who didn't want it, who attacked him. And that is the way of it. Anything that grows and is a success is going to come under greater and greater attack. Now that is a part of the success, succeeding through the struggle. It is a way that eliminates a lot of lesser people and lesser things. It also eliminates some good things, some good people. But it is necessary to not only derive the principle but be able to deal with the practicality of its realization. That can get pretty tough.

Having a new insight, a new technique, or a new technology is therefore not enough, in Phelps's view, to constitute an advance in science. The true scientist must also take on the challenge of convincing his or her peers that there is an advance. The hard work of making the case is almost as important as making the instrument.

Related to the issue of building the technology and convincing others of its value is the issue of receiving credit for this work. For Phelps, this is a particularly sore point: The first article on the PET technique, then called PETT, he felt should have had his name first. Ter-Pogossian, as director of the lab, and perhaps with a different notion of both PET and of scientific progress, insisted on his own name being first. For Phelps, this was not only improper but enough reason to leave the lab and start a new PET program elsewhere (at the University of California, Los Angeles [UCLA]). The blow, he felt, was to his name:

PHELPS: Every development in science is more complicated than some would make it out to be. In fact, it is not necessarily more complicated; it is that there is more to it. Internally in science, we are forced to try and simplify how something happened and who did it. It is not done to ignore what individuals had all contributed to it, but we're forced — by promotions, by awards and prizes in science — to say that this person and this person contributed, but this was the most fundamental contribution. It is an awkward and difficult thing for us to do. But in the end, that is why when you think about DNA you think about Watson and Crick. They didn't collect one piece of data, but there were many people contributing, and they put together the information in a way that made sense that was the double helix. But there are many people contributing.

DUMIT: Yes, that is one of the things I am trying to account for, the many people contributing to this whole development.

PHELPS: Yes. It is an awkward thing to say this contribution is more important than that one, or really to be able to come to the point that you can say that clearly this was more, this was the original idea and from whom it came. It is a tough, tough thing.

The problem that Phelps raises is a common one in science. Many fundamental disagreements in science revolve around credit, and in particular first authorship. Researchers all acknowledge the continual challenge of collaboration. PET's experimental and multidisciplinary nature requires an especially intense attention to these issues. One PET researcher observed the following:

This kind of work requires complete cooperation among people who aren't in the same department. We are all in this together. Despite this grand happy family approach, everyone in academia has to deal with the bottom line, which is first author and intellectual property rights. How do you divide up an experiment that is intrinsically dependent on so many individuals? It is one of the most difficult parts of this endeavor. I think it is one of the reasons why politically there are more problems with PET scanning than many other arenas (although PET is not unique), because you can't do it alone. It is the nature of the beast. Unfortunately, the system of rewards in academia doesn't recognize that you can have six authors and they all participated equally. One person is forced to the front of the line. How do you really convey the degree of contribution? It is tough.

In sum, for Phelps, PET is a watershed information technology. It is a paradigm shift that makes new data available that then has to be championed. Building a working PET device was a crucial technological achievement, and convincing the scientific community that this was so required a difficult marketing practice. In the end, PET enabled new kinds of applied work to be accomplished.

MICHEL M. TER-POGOSSIAN, PH.D.
PET AS FIELD OF RESEARCH, SCIENCE AS NATURAL PROGRESS

With these words in mind, let me now awkwardly turn to Michel M. Ter-Pogossian. Like Phelps, he has also been called the inventor of PET, even "father of PET." I asked him about this:

DUMIT: I saw in one article that you were quoted as being the father of PET. Are there many fathers of PET?

TER-POGOSSIAN: Well, I'm glad that you are saying that. Because when somebody referred to me as the father of PET, I said, "I'd rather be the mother of PET, because many offspring have many fathers, and only one mother. As a matter of fact, some offspring have no father at all!" Of course there are many fathers. And I think that if you look at the first slide that I showed you, [it's obvious that] there are masses of fathers of PET.

Again, the important point is — I'm not suggesting that to you; it is probably obvious — is again the convergence of so many different disciplines. The development of the scintillation counter, artificial radioactivity, and so on. It appears that we are going back pretty far — but you have to go far when doing history — to the radon

41

reconstruction, for instance, which had nothing whatsoever to do with medicine.

Ter-Pogossian's comments reveal a different conception of PET and a different conception of science. Where Phelps highlighted the creative and hard work of tinkering to bring about a practical convergence in the form of a working machine, Ter-Pogossian interpreted an accumulation of thought work, a gene pool rather than a progenitor, an impersonal convergence in place of a triumphant Banister.

The metaphor of convergence, however, does not have the same force epistemologically as a technological innovation. It does not do anything in itself; it does not produce compelling pictures and elegant quantitative information. In Ter-Pogossian's view, PET requires a team on a small scale:

> Well, at that time, we had quite a group of people involved just in general in the utilization of the short-lived radionuclides. We had Michael Welch; we had Mark Raichle; we had two chemists, Michael Phelps and Ed Hoffman, who later on were deeply involved in positron emission tomography. And we had an electronic engineer by the name of Nizar Mullani who continued being interested in the field of positron emission tomography. We were working as a group. All of these people contributed to the development of the probe system that we used and later on configured it indeed to the development of the type of PET devices that we use here. So it was a fairly large group at the time, again, of chemists and physicists. The mathematics contribution came mostly from Biomedical Computing Laboratory, although we all were involved up to a certain degree. So there were a number of people involved. I think it is very important to recognize that it is very much of a team effort.

Ter-Pogossian emphasized that PET is the product of teamwork in the field of short-lived radionuclides. In an early 1981 article defining PET also published in *Seminars in Nuclear Medicine*, Ter-Pogossian described essential areas of work that are integral to PET. He began by noting that the critical components of PET are the physiological properties of the positron-emitting radionuclides. Carbon, nitrogen, and oxygen are common in almost every molecule in our bodies; therefore, tracers using their isotopes can image almost any biologic process.[19]

> A crucial component in the utilization of positron imaging in biology and medicine is the fact that four radionuclides 13N, 15O, and 18F, which possess chemical properties of particular value in biologic investigations, decay with the emission of positrons. . . . It is probable that if it were not for the existence of the above "physiologic" radionuclides, the reconstruction process used in positron emission

tomography would have found little value in biology and in medicine; conversely, the effective utilization in many studies of the "physiologic" radionuclides antedates the PET reconstruction process. (Ter-Pogossian 1981, p. 13)

The core aspect of PET for Ter-Pogossian is the use of the physiological properties that predate the actual PET device. Also, note the impersonality of the historical narrative. PET's value hinges on a coincidence, that positron-emitting nuclides happen to be physiologic ones. These properties were Ter-Pogossian's special area of study from the 1950s onward and were considered to be his triumph over naysayers. In an article on the history of PET, he narrates it this way:

> Between the middle 1940s and the early 1950s, the interest in using 11-C, 13-N, and 18-F in biomedical studies dwindled. . . . For practical purposes, short-lived, cyclotron-produced, positron-emitting radionuclides became inconsequential in biomedical research between the middle 1940s and the middle 1950s, thus ending the first phase of PET.
> In the middle 1950s, Ter-Pogossian and Powers rekindled at Washington University an interest in using, in spite of their short half-lives, short-lived radionuclides for physiological studies. . . . These early experiments stimulated active work with short-lived, cyclotron-reproduced radionuclides, particularly gases, at the Hammersmith Hospital in London. . . . Encouraged by these early results in the decade following the 1960s, the scope of the use of these short-lived physiological radionuclides grew slowly at first. This use then grew more rapidly in a number of centers. . . . (Ter-Pogossian 1992, pp. 142–143)

For Ter-Pogossian, then, PET consisted not of an invention but of a recognition—his noticing that in fact positron emitters would be useful. The pieces of the convergence did not just fall into place anonymously; they had to be recognized as important. In his narrative, science proceeds far more smoothly than in Phelps's; interests are kindled, they stimulate further work, then the work rapidly grows. Science is described as a steady process of work needing an occasional kick, or reorientation, such as when an important path is missed. Indeed, Ter-Pogossian's definition of PET was specifically expanded beyond the scanner:

> Thus, the term "PET" most often encompasses, in addition to the image reconstruction "per se," the utilization of "physiologic" radionuclides. In the context, this definition will be used for PET, and it is useful to emphasize that some facets of the present study would not apply to a narrower definition of the term. (Ter-Pogossian 1981, p. 13)

43

PET, in this view of science, is a path, a path that both includes the convergence of other paths and participates in them. The development of the actual PET scanning device, although necessary, was also inevitable and therefore secondary to the advancement of ways of capitalizing on the central fact of recognition of the value of the short-lived cyclotron-produced, positron-emitting radionuclides. The pains taken here to make clear the scope of PET and the *proper* view of history are worth noting. In the following interview excerpt, Ter-Pogossian restates his position on the definition of PET and on the role of recognition in the advancement of science:

> So this is, in my opinion, the important turning point which led to the development of positron emission tomography. The term *positron emission tomography*, as it is, refers to the tomographic reconstruction process. But I do believe that the most important concept is really the chemical nature of the molecules used. If, for example, the chemical nature of positron emitters did not include oxygen-15, nitrogen-13, carbon-11, and fluorine-18, positron emission tomography would never have been developed. The reason for the development of positron emission tomography was indeed to image these nuclides of physiological importance.
>
> Again, without these four nuclides, nuclear medicine tomography certainly would have existed, because it had been developed in the earlier days by David Kuhl and his coworkers, and as you know, it is widely used [today] in the form of SPECT. But positron emitters — the only reason for using positron emitters is because of the chemical nature of these nuclides which makes them so flexible in physiological experiments. Of course, there is another advantage: There is the emission of annihilation radiation, which allows a much greater precision and sensitivity than in SPECT. So essentially I think the crucial point in positron emission tomography was the — if you want to [call it that] — the recognition of the usefulness of these physiologic nuclides.

Ter-Pogossian's contribution, then, was the rescuing of the once-lost path of exploring the value of physiologic nuclides. His work from the 1950s to the 1970s concerned expanding the uses for these nuclides. To this end, he brought the first cyclotron to be installed in a medical school.[20] Without this path being established, he was saying, there would be no PET:

> There is an amusing aspect from an historical perspective: A number of Nobel laureates have contributed to PET. As far as the discovery of radioactivity is concerned, of course it is Frederic Joliot and Irène Curie. The invention of the cyclotron is Ernest Lawrence. And

as far as the development of tomography, it is Godfried Hounsfield and Allan Cormack. So you see, PET essentially consists of putting together these different building blocks, including all of these areas.

Ter-Pogossian's historical metaphor, then, is not one of obligatory passage points but one of building blocks, with science working slowly, but surely, and steadily down paths.

HENRY N. WAGNER JR., M.D.
PET AS HANDY TOOL, SCIENCE AS CREATIVE INSIGHT

Henry Wagner presents a quite different view on PET. Wagner is a long-standing leader and advocate in the field of nuclear medicine, and his work concentrates on studying neurotransmitters with PET and other nuclear medicine modalities.

The following is an exchange I had with him over the history of PET. Notice how Wagner reframes PET from a technology or technique into a problem that needed solving. In doing so, PET becomes secondary to the scientists who solve primary problems.

DUMIT: I'm working backwards, looking at the history of what are the problems that PET came about to solve. What got these different disciplines together to produce PET?

WAGNER: Good question. How did PET come about? I'll give you some key events. Claude Bernard invented the seeds of the dynamic states of body constituents. Georg [von] Hevesy invented the tracer concept. The cyclotron was used to produce carbon-11, and very interesting studies were done investigating photosynthesis and the metabolism of carbon monoxide. But then, when the reactor got invented and carbon-14 came on the scene, people forgot about the cyclotron because it was too complicated, and they were applying the tracer principle of Hevesy to study the physiological principle of Claude Bernard. The cyclotron was put on the back burner and biochemistry was developing. Okay, then Kety and Sokoloff began making human measurements; they began studying brain blood flow. And they began studying brain blood flow and behavior in a global sense. And they tried to study things like schizophrenia and anesthesia and things like that. And they carried out some studies using radioactive tracers to measure global blood flow. Then a parallel path was imaging, which began basically with the thyroid, studying regional function of organs such as the thyroid gland, and imaging was being developed. And [Sokoloff's group], they were trying to show some brain chemical process going on in association with activation, and they used autoradiography to show that you could stimulate a cat and get an activation in the brain. This turned everybody on. Then chance came into the picture—chance plays a tremendous role in all of these things. By chance, Martin Reivich was working at the NIH with Sokoloff and Kety, and he went up to Pennsylvania, where they had a nuclear medicine guy, David Kuhl. They then said, "We are going to extend the autoradiographic studies of Sokoloff to human beings." And that is exactly what we did here [at Johns Hopkins University]. I saw the autoradiograph studies of Michael Kuhar and said, "We are going to translate that into human studies."

So PET arose to translate the autoradiograph studies of Kety and Sokoloff to human beings. That was the event. These things are obviously a chain reaction, but every now and then you get an event where you can put a mark at that particular event. That event was the Kety and Sokoloff part [italics mine].

Now you are saying that this is different. [But] there [with Kety and Sokoloff] is a problem! They said that there is some chemical process going on in your brain, electrical activity is related to behavior, they wanted to relate chemistry to behavior. That's the problem. Why did you say that you are working in the opposite direction?

DUMIT: The stories that I have seen of PET, described in articles and so on, describe PET as the product of a number of technical achievements such as computers, small cyclotrons, new tracer methods. These things came on the scene and people were basically waiting for new things to happen such as new algorithms. When this happened, then . . .

WAGNER: That is ridiculous. I don't understand. There is a series of events that happened, and these events all went in that direction. I don't understand how people were waiting for something to happen. What were they doing while they were waiting? They were sitting there waiting—for someone to open up the door and announce something?

DUMIT: A stopping point.

WAGNER: No, that is not true. Research is based on taking the instruments. . . . I read a really good description, in a history of neurosciences written by Hodgkin, and he pointed out that discoveries are made by curious people who use the equipment that is available at the time, and they will find out something based on almost any equipment that is present. And major discoveries were made using unbelievably primitive equipment. So the idea that somebody's sitting there waiting for something to be invented, some measuring device to be invented to solve their problem, is not correct. What you have are parallel paths and inventions. And long before we had these inventions, computers, people were doing tomography. I mean Dave Kuhl did back-projection in 1963. I mean, it depends. It is a continuum, and every now and then something is so outstanding it sort of stands out, but it is a continuum. Let's say you have a coming together of all these things. I mean, PET would not be in the state that it is today if it had not been for parallel developments that were happening. So to say that people were waiting for it to happen is malarkey. Creative people were making the best use — pure science is creative, curious people making do with what they have, beginning with their eyes. Darwin had his eyeballs. Isn't that right? He wasn't waiting around for computers to be developed, the tracer principle to be invented.

Claude Bernard was not sitting there waiting for the tracer principle to carry out his studies. He was trying to do an impossible thing; he was making an observation. It takes a curious person to solve a problem. So PET was a chain of events. So two absolutely outstanding people in it were Bernard and Hevesy, then there were regional measurements made of the thyroid gland. Thyroid scanning started because of nodules in the thyroid. They wanted to know whether they were functional or not functional; they had a spatial problem.

For Wagner, science follows problems. Science progresses because there are creative thinkers who struggle with practical problems, medical problems. Neither part of the Phelps–Ter-Pogossian difference (technological invention or path recognition) succeeds in *propelling* science. They are valuable sideshows to the progress of thinkers. Wagner's history might be represented as paradigms shifting by insights.

The significance of problems with both instrument and nuclides is best illustrated in the following comment, in which Wagner refocused my interest in PET onto the kinds of problems and domains with which he is working.[21]

In fact, I really don't distinguish between PET and SPECT as being two different things. It's just a question of different tracers. Everything is the same except the tracers. So basically, some of the biggest advances in cancer were not with a PET agent but with a SPECT agent that is a gross suppresser substance. And we know that many cancers are associated with an increase in somatostatin receptors, where somatostatin is something that tells cells to stop secreting and stop dividing. When you find an up-regulation, or an increase in the receptor, you look for a deficiency in the messenger. And that's what it's turning out to be in the case [of] certain brain tumors. For example, there is a deficiency in the production of a chemical that tells cells to stop secreting and stop dividing. So all cancer [research] is being transformed into a molecular approach; it is being defined in a molecular domain.

In one fell swoop, in one sweeping sentence, Wagner's view of the problem of PET sidesteps the views of both Phelps and Ter-Pogossian: "I really don't distinguish between PET and SPECT as being two different things." The crucial components of each of their claims appear interchangeable with other components—Phelps's scanner for SPECT, Ter-Pogossian's physiological positron emitters for single-photon nuclides. Neither was crucial. They were important, maybe, but not critical, and certainly not obligatory. Wagner is not interested in the mechanics of the tools, though he knows them. Instruments are tools whose purpose is to vanish into the background of science. The question of PET tracers he hears as one about tracers in general, which is part of the solution to a problem about cancer, which in turn is about thinking through the process of cellular communication and growth.

So . . . Toward a Historiography of PET

Represented in these three individuals are three kinds of deterministic histories—technology, scientific principles, scientific research. PET is either a critical invention, a crucial application of an insight, or one among many tools at hand.

What is a historian to do with all this? If I follow Wagner (my particular abstraction of Wagner), then a history of PET is not even a true project. I might write a history of the solution to the problem of autoradiography in humans, perhaps, but in any case, it would be a history of ideas and insights, with politics and political economy entering only to provide color and chance.

To adopt Phelps's perspective, on the contrary, would be to focus on political economy and politics, the day-to-day specifics of how work actually gets done or gets suppressed in institutions. A Phelpsian history would highlight the hard work not only of creatively making something work, but also of marketing it, and where marketing would mean not only demonstrating that it works effectively but also convincing others of this effectiveness. Paradigms would be shown to be the result of lobbying as much as of insight.

Ter-Pogossian's perspective would also involve political economy, but not as much politics. A scientific history would require attending to directions in science, to insightful proposals for research, and directions

48

lost and regained. It would highlight an army of tireless, careful researchers but also attend to skill in promoting research directions and building programs with vision.

Each of these historiographical approaches raises fundamental questions about the definition and purpose of both PET and of science. Each also would highlight different kinds of documents and emphasize different people. Like many websites on the Internet, the history of PET is "still under construction."

DUMIT: I was just thinking of functional images. I am still working
at understanding how a function, or something that happens
through time, is represented in a PET picture. Because it looks like
one instant in time, [like a photograph], even though for most PET
pictures it is two minutes, maybe twenty minutes.

TER-POGOSSIAN: Sure, but that is not the important portion at all.

DUMIT: What would you say is the important portion?

TER-POGOSSIAN: It is the function itself. And the function itself is
again derived through the application of a physiological model,
which is certainly not instantaneous at all. In some cases, the instantaneous image is perfectly all right. Let me give you a specific
case: the accumulation of FDG in a brain tumor. Well, that is an
instantaneous phenomenon. But if you are trying to measure actually the glucose metabolism by FDG, an instantaneous picture
really is not going to give you anything. I mean you have to take a
series of measurements, you have to plug into measurements blood
activities, and very often reconstruct a completely different image
from the one that you obtained instantaneously, taking into account the other factors.

DUMIT: With the oxygen studies, it is the same thing.

TER-POGOSSIAN: Yes. The image itself doesn't show anything. In fact,
we often don't show the images. You show an image if you want to
show the morphology [anatomical structure] in a given portion of
the heart. And put a square and put a number, and that number
indicates the bloodflow in that portion of the myocardium, which

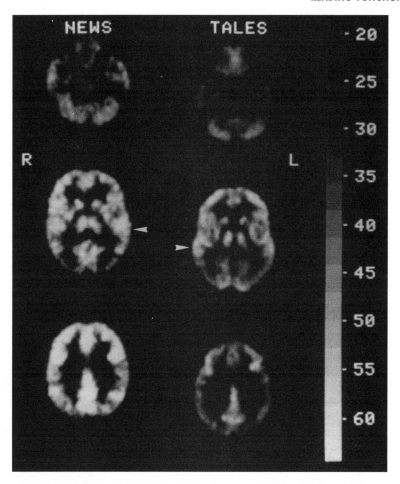

FIGURE 2.1. News versus tales. Original caption reads: "Typical corresponding cerebral glucose metabolism (μmol/100 g. per minute) PET images of normal right-handers during verbal auditory stimulation, with one listening to interesting news and the other to boring tales, showing differential activation and lateralization of Wernicke's area response (*arrowheads*)." (Pawlik and Heiss 1989)

is calculated on the basis of a series of images, as a matter of fact, plus the blood activity. And the blood activity in cardiac studies is usually taken out of one of the ventricles.

But in certain cases, indeed you have purely morphological images. The FDG accumulation in a brain tumor is purely morphological [because they are interested not in *how fast* the tumor accumulates FDG but only in the anatomical location of the tumor that accumulates

51

FDG much faster than any other area in the brain]. That is not the strength of PET.

DUMIT: Activation images, though, would be kind of in between?

TER-POGOSSIAN: Activation images [figure 2.1] are in between; you are right. But you see an activation image—really, to interpret an activation image, you really have to calculate the flow, and the calculation of the flow is a dynamic process. That is probably, incidentally, the reason for the relative difficulty in interpreting PET images. The complexity—perhaps not the difficulty—is something that has slowed down the development of PET. In clinical practice you don't like to do that at all. And for very good reasons: You don't have time for that.

DUMIT: Because it takes a lot more time to go through and make sure the physiological [parameters and calculations are correct]?

TER-POGOSSIAN: Well, yes. It requires all the measurements, the blood activity as a function of time. That means you have to take samples in some way and measure the samples. And then you have to sit down with a computer and apply a model of some sort to make sense out of that. It is much easier to look at a picture and say, "You know, it is right there." That is not the way you do things in PET.

That is not completely true, because under certain circumstances that is just what you do. . . . Let me put it this way: If I look at an image, or at numbers, I am more concerned with *what* it represents than *how* it represents it. I don't know whether that answers your question. But I am trying. When I see a hot area on an image or a series of numbers, I try to think of whether it is an accumulation, or whether it is an inert process of some sort occurring, whether it is necrotic tissue-absorbing activity. Yes, in general, this is what stimulates my thinking.

DUMIT: So images or numbers—it doesn't matter; it is the process. . . .

TER-POGOSSIAN: It is the process, yes, underlying it.

Chapter 3
Producing Brain Images of Mind

We know we need hype to sell our research; let's try to keep it out of the results!
— Louis Sokoloff, giving a plenary talk at a Society for Neuroscience national meeting

PET researchers are clearly torn between conflicting visions of PET. A part of each researcher wants to impress the world with the great progress made in discovering the brain's functions as well with his or her own great mastery of the complexity of the brain. Another part wants the world to know how difficult this task is, how many assumptions and equipment limitations have to be carefully balanced, and how tricky pulling off a successful experiment actually is. But the most compelling desire of each PET researcher is to turn off all of this world concern and just dive into the exciting mysteries of the brain, using this fascinating, innovative, challenging technology. Understanding a PET experiment requires understanding how these three desires of the PET researcher are carried out together in every experiment and in every publication.

Coming to a deeper understanding of the mind–brain relationship is why many neuroscientists went into science in the first place. From the technological perspective, the brain is a seriously difficult nut to crack. It is protected by a skull, it is unimaginably complex and interconnected (100,000 neurons in a cubic millimeter), and all of these neurons and synapses are going about their business at the same time. Therefore, for potential researchers looking for insight into the brain at work, functional brain imaging offered an unbelievable opportunity: to extract information otherwise impossible to get from a living brain while correlating this information with the activity of the person. Peter Fox described, in an interview, the thirst for knowledge:

> I was in medical school [in the 1970s, and] that was at the time that the *Scientific American* article came out . . . showing brain mapping with xenon blood flow [see Plate 10] techniques in Denmark. . . . For four years in a row, I [had been working on] a thesis on epistemology and wanted to know how the brain lets us know how it is we perceive the world, and how the brain is organized to allow us to have knowledge of our environment. And it was immediately apparent, [as] people were mapping this and arguing at that stage about the role of SMA [supplementary motor area] and how high a processor it was . . . at any rate, at that time people were getting very excited by it, and it was clear that you could map the brain. I was debating at that time whether to go into psychiatry or neurology, and at that point, seeing the emergence of brain mapping techniques, decided to go into neurology.

We can point to the rise of PET technology in the mid-1970s, but the development of PET is still ongoing in the twenty-first century. A short list of the disciplines involved in PET experiments include physicists, chemists, nuclear chemists, biologists, computer scientists, electrical engineers, psychologists, psychiatrists, neurologists, oncologists, nuclear medicine specialists, neuroanatomists, mathematicians. These specialists must cooperate extensively with each other to understand how each area of expertise depends on the results of everyone else's areas, as a senior researcher said to me:

> The thing with all of PET scanning is that it is an unusual kind of research, because it requires intense collaborative participation from people from very diverse scientific viewpoints. Usually in science, you're a physiologist or you're an anatomist; you are in a lab, you have your experiment, all nicely and neatly self-contained. For the most part you don't *need* direct participation from disciplines that are removed from what you do (although collaborations across related disciplines are common), whereas the most successful PET labs have been those that have been able to capitalize on the symbiosis of very diverse groups of investigators — chemists, physicists, theoretical modelers, clinicians, neuroscientists, psychologists, linguists, etc. The boss needs to facilitate the interaction of scientists who have little to no training in specific brain mechanisms [and] clinicians or behaviorists who may have no clue about the intricacies of the technology. PET

requires the close cooperation of people who ordinarily would have no reason to interact with one another in a research endeavor. No one person can do it without the others.

At a recent Society of Nuclear Medicine meeting, for instance, papers were presented by physicists and mathematicians proposing new architectures for scanners, new compounds for detector crystals, and new algorithms for better correction of errors in reconstruction. Chemists presented work on better radioligands to specify more precisely what the brain is doing during scans. Tasks were critiqued by psychiatrists, neurologists, and psychologists. Patient-selection procedures, scan resolution, and statistical analysis were all subject to intense scrutiny. Indeed, there were no aspects within the entire PET apparatus that were not contested or shown to be contestable.

At the same time, there were specific results presented for neurological, psychiatric, psychological, cardiological, and oncological studies done with PET. In order to evaluate the meaning of the results, the presenters pragmatically had to act as if their PET apparatus worked unproblematically. Each individual researcher is often limited in the aspects of the experiment he or she can critique or even follow. Paper presenters are often asked questions to which their response is: "I'm not sure; another researcher handled that part of the experiment." Whether these presenters are psychiatrists who do not know how the brain images were normalized to a "reference brain," or chemists who are not sure how normal control patients were chosen, or computer scientists who do not know how specifically the radiopharmaceutical binds to a particular receptor, questions are often left hanging and questioners are left frustrated by their inability to deconstruct the presented data into data relevant to their own interests.

Another downside of PET's complexity and requisite cooperation is that each expert participant is also responsible for a successful career path, publications, leadership, and credit. Thus, despite the practical achievement of complex cooperation in PET in many centers, disputes still arise over the ultimate meaning and usefulness of the data, both among labs and between groups of researchers at the same lab. Often, different groups within the same center use PET in paradigmatically different ways, and they find it difficult to communicate with each other.

DUMIT: I have wondered if there has been a tension in PET between the image as qualitative and the image as quantitative. PET seems to be a great difference engine. It can produce a difference between different kinds of people or different kinds of traits and states.

PHELPS: Yes. Of course, part of that is also conflict built into PET, in that there are many different people involved in PET. There are

55

conflicts between those who use it qualitatively and superficially and those who use it analytically, by their nature. There can be people who are trying to use it to do some clinical research, or deal with the limitations in people. You know you can't be doing their biochemistry by other techniques, pulling out their tissue and analyzing it. So the paradigms, the research paradigms, are quite different. So they can be exploring the relationship between the brain and behavior in the domain that they normally work in. And the basic neurochemist involved in PET will say, "I don't like that; you don't know what you are talking about. What are the units of your data, depression on this axis versus color on this axis?" So there are a lot of different factions within PET, because it does go from basic chemists and biologists to clinical investigators, and their criteria of an experiment are quite different.

Each of these stages involves both necessary assumptions about persons and brains, and in many experiments each part of the experimental process is being innovated and tested at the same time. In the same experiment, then, a physicist may be testing a hypothesis regarding a new scanner architecture, a pharmacologist may be testing a hypothesis regarding the action of a drug on a speech impediment, a neurologist may be testing where in the brain the speech impediment is "located," and a computer scientist may be testing a new algorithm for defining significant locations in averaged brain scans. Such an experiment requires a degree of interdisciplinary cooperation uncommon in research. It is a delicate balancing act in which each hypothesis can be tested only by assuming that the other hypotheses are not significant to one's results.

Another senior researcher described how these different research agendas can coexist around the same machine:

We never really had a very structured system. But each one of these subgroups, and you know we had subgroups, developed their own interests, and they developed their own grants. So little by little, we had a series of PET subgroups, or groups, working relatively harmoniously together, but not specifically as one monolithic institute in the European sense of the word. As a matter of fact, this balkanization of PET, certainly in our institution, is very strong now. There really is a whole series of subgroups working on their own, with their own ideas. They are on good terms with other people and from time to time seek help or give help. But otherwise they have their own source of funding and their own interests. The cardiologists very seldom talk to the neurologists. This is not out of any kind of dislike; they just have their own interests. PET has become something a little bit like a microscope, if you will. And the chemists also have their own interests. They spend their time making more and more complicated molecules and labeling them in specific positions.

The ability of PET researchers to work together is crucial, and yet sharing credit is a continual source of tension. Being the first author on published articles is the most prestigious.[1] For an experiment that tests a new scanner with a new radioligand on patients with a psychiatric illness, for instance, the leading psychiatrist, chemist, and physicist often will each present a paper at different disciplinary conferences and/or publish an article in different journals. However, this practice of multiplying first-authorship is not perfect, and credit remains a difficult issue, especially as domains of responsibility shift.[2]

Although this necessary cooperation may be a source of great concern and frustration of PET researchers, it is ironically one of the reasons why they like the field so much. "I was bored doing organic chemistry," said one chemistry researcher, "With PET, you have to know so much more about what is going on, it is exciting." Another chemist concurred and emphasized the increased significance his discipline has within PET: "PET is probably one of the few fields where chemists have sway over the M.D.'s. If they don't respect you, you don't give them isotope!" As we will see, the same increased significance is true for each specialist in a PET experiment. They all become vital to the success of the experiment. In other words, each person is responsible to a whole consisting of many experts who are each not just important but critical to the final production and interpretation of data.

Despite this profound interdisciplinary complexity, brain-imaging data is presented in a particularly simple and compelling manner: PET images appear to be discrete, readable, and colorful. Similarly, because the process appears to produce clean pictures of functional brain activity, many simple diagrams of the PET process have been displayed as shorthand illustrations of it. Figure 1.1 makes PET seem almost as simple and as automatic as taking a snapshot. This leads not only to enthusiasm for brain imaging but to misplaced recruitment as well, as one researcher explained:

> It is kind of funny: I have had many people express an interest in using PET, typically established scientists in many fields who may be on a downhill curve of their career. Very overtly they express that PET is such a high road to science that they're willing to get involved now. They kind of held back before, but now they are willing to get involved because it is obviously so easy! They lack an understanding of what is entailed, I think, because the data comes out as pretty pictures. You put up these slides that show the brain turning on and

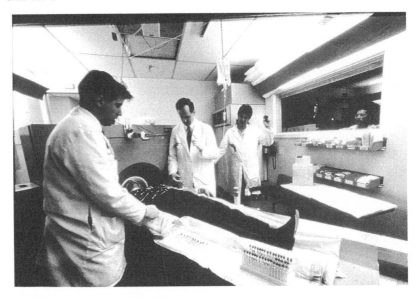

FIGURE 3.1. PET procedure in progress at Johns Hopkins University Medical Center. A research doctor, assisted by two technicians in the room and another one in the computer room behind shielded glass, draws blood and monitors the patient. (Marcus 1995)

turning off. They just don't understand the work that is involved in making these experiments happen.

It is crucial, therefore, to unpack the kind of complexity required to produce and understand PET images (Figure 3.1) as well as to understand the social function and efficacy of such simple diagrams.

The remainder of this chapter examines how the data produced in a PET experiment is visualized as an image of a living brain slice, and how those images are produced in the lab, selected, and published to make meaningful, factual claims about the world. My thesis is that the visuality of these images, their apparent familiarity, and their transparency with regard to the brain all contribute to the potency of PET claims. PET researchers have acknowledged the difficulty of properly producing and understanding these images, and have warned that "we must understand our tools before we can hope to understand our results" (Perlmutter and Raichle 1986). I am arguing that the processes of producing, selecting, and presenting images in both scientific articles and in public arenas require the same sort of understanding.

Creating Experiments: A Difficult Task

Creating experiments based on this work demands a tremendous team effort. The first thing one realizes when entering a PET lab is that the scanner is only one piece of a large-scale technical system. Technical descriptions of the scanning process only begin to define the work of conducting an actual experiment, however; they describe the stage and players, but not the play. Heuristically, we can break the whole process into four stages: design, measure, manipulate, and visualize.

1. Experiment design: The first stage of the process involves choosing participants for the study and designing their state and behavior in the scanner. Defining criteria for participant inclusion requires delimiting the boundaries of "normal human" for purposes of the study. Is a chronic smoker or coffee drinker normal enough? How about someone who had been found to have depression 10 years ago and has taken Prozac for 6 months — or someone whose brother is schizophrenic? Likewise, if the study is comparing two groups, the experimental group must also be characterized.

Because the purpose of the scan is to detect brain function, every part of the person's state of mind and brain needs to be controlled for. This includes what each subject eats or drinks beforehand, how rested or anxious the subject is, and what exactly the subject does inside the scanner. The more precise the state can be defined and calibrated, the easier it will be to compare results with those of other experiments.

2. Measuring brain activity: The second stage covers the scanning process proper. The radioactive molecules must be prepared and then injected into the person. The scanner must properly collect the data, and then a computer must algorithmically reconstruct the data into a three-dimensional map of activity, based on assumptions about the scanner and brain activity. The result is a dataset keyed to the individual's brain activity, a brainset.

3. Making data comparable: In stage 3, the individual brainsets are transformed and normalized so that the individual's brain locations can be correlated with those of others. With the use of MRI data and digital brain atlases, anatomical areas corresponding to the brainset can be found. Next, different brainsets can be combined and checked for statistical significance using subtraction, averaging, and other forms of data set manipulation. The result is a collective group brainset.

4. Making comparable data presentable: Finally, in stage 4, the brainsets are made visible. First, colors are used to substitute for the numbers in the dataset, and second, specific colored brainsets are selected to be

produced and published. Coloring involves transforming numeric variation into a contour map, highlighting some differences at the expense of
others.

Turning then to the postproduction events for images, particular images are selected for publication and presented in journals. At the heart
of this process is a common, standard, and often encouraged practice of
selecting extreme images. This is an acknowledged, troubling practice,
necessary for scientific work and yet increasingly problematic as these
images travel outside of expert circles and into popular culture, where
new, less-qualified labels are applied.

Each of the stages and substeps within them is hotly debated, and
along the way there are many assumptions about human anatomy,
human physiology, and human nature. As discussed above, however,
rather than exploding the coherence of the PET experiment, each assumption can become the grounds for a different discipline's article. The
complexity and theory-ladenness of the PET experiment is thus incredibly productive of scientific results.

STAGE 1: EXPERIMENTAL DESIGN

Subject Selection and Injection

A senior PET researcher described subject selection:

> Collaboration is fine. Share data, collaborate, talk about it, work it
> out. But just having it in a base where somebody can pull it out, I
> think, creates a lot of chaos. One of the difficulties is [that] too many
> people have access to the databases and can make changes that you
> would never know about. So when I go for normal controls, I go to
> our normal control database, but I have to be very careful going
> through it. Just because they are labeled normal controls doesn't
> mean they are. I tend to use normal controls that I have generated
> myself in my own studies. I don't take the ones generated in other
> people's studies in the same group, because I don't really know what
> they did. But I don't think that that is a major impediment to the
> science.

Choosing people to be scanned for a study can be one of the most
difficult procedures. In extreme cases, such as finding schizophrenics
who are drug-naive (who have never taken medication or illegal drugs),
the work of actually locating and validating proper subjects can constitute grounds for claiming first authorship on the published article! The
problem, as I have come to understand it, involves group and individual
definition of variability and constraint: To what extent is an individual

representative of a group, and to what extent is the group well-characterized? These problems are exacerbated or exaggerated because PET often involves very small study sizes (four to twenty subjects) because of cost, radioactivity, and time constraints, and because PET often provides information for which there is no independent verification. This means that often the only way to corroborate the findings of PET study is with another PET study. There is no easy end to possible confounding variables.

Because there was no other way to verify the data that PET produces, one of the first tasks of PET researchers was to characterize normals (Mazziotta and et al. 1981; Mazziotta and Phelps 1985; Raichle 1994a). Only then could non-normals be compared. However, creating a baseline definition of normals is both a physiological and a social judgment. The following description provides a list of the tests used to characterize persons as normals in one study:

> The normal population consisted of 20 males aged 19–59 years. Inclusion in the study was determined by the absence of medical, neurological, and psychological pathology. Medical reasons for exclusion were a history of severe head trauma, chronic hypertension, significant vascular disorders, diabetes mellitus, thyroid abnormalities, and a history of psychiatric illness. Gross psychopathology was identified with the Structured Clinical Interview (SCI), an inventory of 17 yes-or-no items filled out by the examiner during a 20- to 30-min. interview. The SCI can also be scored for 13 overlapping scales: anger, hostility, conceptual dysfunction, fear, worry, incongruous behavior, incongruous ideation, lethargy, dejection, perceptual dysfunction, physical complaints, self-depreciation, and sexual problems. Any score significantly beyond the norms on any SCI component automatically excluded the candidate. Neurological and neurophysiological screening included medical history and testing for intelligence (WAIS [Wechsler Adult Intelligence Scale]), anterograde memory [Randt-NYU Memory Test (Randt 1980)], perceptual-motor function and structure (Bender Visual-Motor Gestalt Test), and handedness [Edinburgh Handedness Inventory (Oldfield 1971)]. Subjects also underwent a comprehensive laboratory work-up, a brief neurological screening examination, CT (to provide scans which could be correlated with PETT), computerized EEG [electroencephalography], and testing of visual and auditory evoked potentials (John et al. 1977). (Brodie et al. 1983, p. 201)

The tremendous amount of work put into finding such "normal" subjects was done with the intent of avoiding "noise" in the resulting data. Georges Canguilhem's book *The Normal and the Pathological* traces the history of the terms *normal*, *abnormal*, *pathological*, and *anoma-lous* through various sciences and medicines. Canguilhem noted that *normal* has been a polyvalent term that in different texts meant "typ-ically healthy" (what the patient desires to be), "quantitatively aver-age," "not anomalous," or "ideal" (in the sense of being not at all pathological or unhealthy) (Canguilhem 1978). Medical characteriza-tions of diseases are historically defined from a therapeutic perspective; one is diseased if one is not typically healthy and seeks therapeutic care. Initial studies with brain images are based on selections of "ideal" sub-jects, or "supernormals" who have no probable pathology.

> Normal age-matched controls have been studied in conjunction with this project. Healthy controls best consist of persons selected to minimize the possibility of covert pathology. These so-called 'super-normals' are individuals who have been observed to be symptom-free for a number of years, have no personal or family history of psychi-atric disorders, and are not users of substances known to influence mood. (Phelps and Mazziotta 1985, p. 459)

The complexity of the project is part of the difficulty of mental-illness research and psychological research in general. Directly measuring the brain adds an additional factor. Possible confounders remain: Are men sufficiently different from women to study separately, or are they suffi-ciently similar to women so that they can be averaged together?[3] Such characteristics as age, ethnicity, handedness, culture (refugee status), sexuality, familial histories, past head trauma, and medical history are all still unknown confounders raised as questions in meetings during presentation of results.

PET brain studies almost always use right-handed male subjects, un-less gender is specifically being studied or a disease is being studied that is significantly more prevalent in females than in males. Although the reasons for this exclusion — cleaner data because of the lack of possible interference from gender or handedness differences — "may be viewed as practical from a financial standpoint, it results in . . . a lack of informa-tion about the etiology of some diseases in women" (Rosser 1994).[4] By choosing only men for these studies, the researchers implicitly assume that gender matters. But by treating the results of the experiments as applicable to normal humans in general, they risk the consequence that a gender difference may appear as an abnormality.

For large-scale studies of schizophrenia, with over fifty people being studied, race is often recorded, though not consistently. In PET studies where the extreme expense of the procedure and the time involved re-sults in very small samples, typically between four and twenty, race has almost never been mentioned. Analogous to the circumstances for gender, the assumption is that there probably are significant population differences in brain chemistry and anatomy between different races. To eliminate this potentially confounding variable, however, race is often excluded from the sample altogether by using only whites. Financially, for the experimenters, this is the only course of action that makes sense.[5]

Even once these lifelong or *trait* characteristics are accounted for, temporary or *state* characteristics remain. For some studies, normals are only those who have not had caffeine that day.[6] Use of nicotine, vitamins, or other drugs must also be monitored. Debates go on about proper cooling-off periods for drugs and medication. Also, questions remain as to the value of "normal databases" based on such exclusionary definitions of normal.

Because there are so many different definitions of normal, of who could be included as a normal control, and how explicitly their attributes should be noted, attempts to standardize a database have so far failed (see Beaulieu 2000 for more).

At the 1995 meeting of the Society of Nuclear Medicine, a new confounder was introduced: One lab reported that the *time of day* during which the scan took place significantly and regionally affected PET results (Diehl and Mintun 1995). This means that a scan taken of a person in the morning, when compared with a scan of the same person taken under the same conditions but in the afternoon, might show a difference in certain areas of the brain and not others. The authors suggested that time-of-day differences might account for specific differences among labs. Certainly, this finding adds to the difficulty of replicating PET findings.

Yet, because the assumption behind this decision to exclude population differences is that these differences probably matter, the production of generically unmarked images with labels such as *normal* and *schizophrenic* (rather than, e.g., *white U.S. right-handed male schizophrenics*) means that we should assume that nonwhites will probably not look normal.[7] When we combine this analysis with the practice of choosing "extreme" images for publication (where normal is chosen because it is farthest away from that particular group of subjects with schizophrenia), we can see yet another reason why the nonsampled nonwhite could more easily be found to be not normal.

Task Design (Types of Scans and Confounders)

Once the subjects have been selected, they must be injected with the radioisotope. What the subjects do or think, once injected, makes task-selection fundamental to the PET data produced, even when the task is not the object of the study. This is one area where PET is completely different from CT or MRI, which image structure. Structure does not change from moment to moment. PET scanning maps rates of flows of molecules in the brain over a relatively small period of time. Consequently, correctly characterizing and understanding a person's behavior, mood, and cognitive activity is essential to understanding the meaning of the flows.

Once injected with the radiotracer, the patient is now "on display." His or her body is emitting radioactivity. During this time, especially for brain studies, what the patient does — moving, thinking, hearing — bears greatly on the final PET scan data. For instance, one classic study compared *seeing* words versus *hearing* words. During the seeing-words task, subjects watched video screens where words were flashed up. During the hearing-words study, subjects listened to different words. PET has proved to be sensitive to different cognitive activities, and discovering the regional differences in brain activity during these activities is often the aim of these studies.

Even if the aim of the study is to characterize disease states, however, the behavior of the subjects still must be controlled for. "Resting" turns out to be a complicated task (Mazziotta et al. 1981). Should one rest with eyes closed or open? With ears blocked, in silence, or listening to music? Does having an injection in one arm focus attention there? Anxiety has been studied, for instance, in part because the PET scan procedure itself might cause anxiety (e.g., at being motionless in a scanner for 30 minutes or being injected with a radioactive substance) (Reiman 1988; Reiman et al. 1989; Wu et al. 1991). Anxiety levels are usually measured before and after studies. With PET, in other words, one is always performing a task[8] (Figure 3.2). Baseline states are all confounding variables to consider in designing a task to be studied.

Depending on the half-life of the tracer used, the subject will carry out the task either before getting into the scanner or while strapped inside. With FDG, for example, the critical uptake time is the first 40 minutes after injection. During this time, the brain traps almost all of the radiotracer in different cells and keeps it there, emitting radioactivity, for about another hour. After the 40 minutes, the subject is placed in the scanner and a picture of the trapped, still-radioactive glucose analog is taken. With oxygen, which has a 2-minute half-life, the subject must already be in the scanner when injected. Scans are performed during the first 2 to 5 minutes, while the subject is performing the task.

Task design is itself one of the most active areas of studies. Studies include cognitive task comparisons (looking at words), states comparisons (such as anxiety or sadness, or cued-state studies such as showing cocaine addicts a video of drug use), resting trait comparisons (patients with Huntington's disease vs. those without it), task–trait comparisons

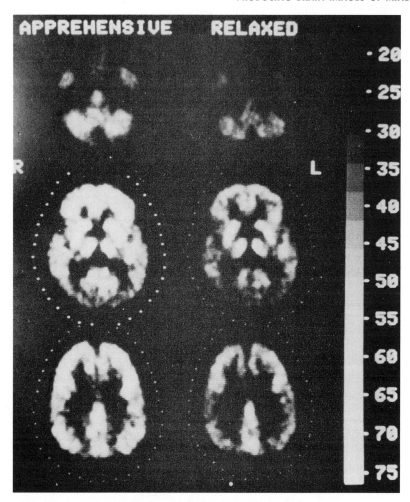

FIGURE 3.2. Apprehensive versus relaxed. Original caption reads: "Matching cerebral glucose metabolism (μmol/100 g per minute) PET images of a healthy, 71-year-old man in apprehensive versus relaxed resting state, eyes closed, ears unoccluded." (Pawlik and Heiss 1989)

(patients with schizophrenia who are hallucinating versus at rest[9]), neurotransmitter binding studies (dopamine, serotonin, etc.), and challenge studies (where a drug is given and the brain's reaction to it is studied). The key problem in designing a particular study of any one of these types (table 3.1) is finding a way to keep the other types from interfering.[10]

Most PET tasks are in the tradition of cognitive psychology or

Table 3.1
Dimensions of Scanning Experiments

Individual activity *or* Group property
Variability in activity *or* Shared properties
Current state of person *or* Long-term trait
"Normal" activity *or* Condition (disease or life stage)
Acute Condition *or* Nonacute Condition
Condition at rest *or* Challenged by task or drug
Duration of scan (2–30 minutes)

cognitive neuroscience (see Plates 5 and 6). The assumption in these tasks is that complex mental functions are the aggregation of simpler component operations. In designing a PET experiment, then, "the control state and the stimulated state are carefully chosen to isolate, as far as possible, a single mental operation" (Raichle 1990).[11] Articles often begin with this assumption of discrete modules or components, each responsible for a different type of cognitive activity. For instance:

Since the brain consists of large numbers of interconnected substructures, damage to one structure or its interconnecting fiber bundles will also result in functional effects at multiple sites throughout any given network. PET has revealed this distributed organization, leading to a more comprehensive view of human functional brain systems in health and disease. (Phelps and Mazziotta 1985)[12]

For cognitive neuroscientists, used to large sample sizes, PET added a new challenge: how to control for as many dimensions of variability as possible. A simple-sounding task like recognizing words might reveal a host of confounding variables, each correlating with a different set of brain regions: the size of the displayed words (how much of the visual field is consumed in the recognition process), the brightness of the word, the rate of presentation (which in fact turned out to produce very different brain activations), the language of the word (is a more ideographic language like Chinese processed differently from English?),[13] educational level, effects on attention, novelty and learning. (Are there effects from simply having to repeat a very simple task over and over that are different from purposeful recognition of words? Is proofreading a different activity from reading?) — these are in addition to designing the series of tasks so that a particularly desired component of language is being isolated. *If* the underlying presumption of modularity is correct *and* the task correctly isolates the component simple mental operation, *then* "from such data emerges a map of the distributed modular organization of the brain underlying normal human cognition and emotion" (Raichle 1990).

There are debates in psychology over whether the modularity hypothesis itself can be tested with PET at all, or whether it must just be assumed.[14] Philosopher Jerry Fodor summarized one of the issues as a very serious struggle over limited resources and the value of different lines of questioning:

> I quite see why anyone who cares how the mind works might reasonably care about the argument between empiricism and rationalism; and why anyone who cares about the argument between empiricism and rationalism might reasonably care whether different areas of the brain differ in the mental functions they perform. . . . But given that it matters to both sides whether, by and large, mental functions have characteristic places in the brain, why should it matter to either side where the places are? . . . what is the question about the mind–brain relation in general, or about language in particular, that turns on where the brain's linguistic capacities are? And if, as I suspect, none does, why are we spending so much time and money trying to find them? (Fodor 1999)[15]

Another form of dispute concerns the significance of individual variability. PET researcher Richard Haier calls himself an "individual differences psychologist," which means he is interested specifically in tasks for which people differ in their performance.[16] If this is the case, then he can look for a correlation between performance and some brain measure. He begins by comparing his work to cognitive psychology.

HAIER: You know what cognitive psychologists do? They ask you to press a button when you see an *M* or an *N*. Either it is presented in this visual field or that visual field. They use very simple stimuli to get at complex processes. The idea of using something like Raven's Advanced Matrices[17] is just outrageous. Even the idea of individual differences in cognitive psychology is not a very big idea. Cognitive psychologists almost by definition are not interested in individual differences.

DUMIT: They are interested in how people share certain characteristics.

HAIER: That is right. So the variance in people's reaction times is regarded as error variance by cognitive psychologists. They want a task that minimizes that. They don't want a task that has a wide range of performance, they want everyone to do about the same, so they can discover "the" process. We took a completely different point of view. It is not that our point of view is better or worse — it is just a different starting point. This is common in psychology.

67

Haier is describing yet another dimension of brain function. In this "individual differences" dimension, humans vary in their performances on tasks and in their brain activation during performances. Video game experiments, for instance, use a task that people got better at. Most PET studies in the last twenty years have minimized this dimension, concentrating on tasks presumed to be relatively similar in performance and brain activity across humans and in time.

In sum, during the design stage, the basic terms of human nature are already built into the experiment. Subject selection defines a concept of the normal human being in the form of an ideal (super)normal. Abnormal categories, such as mental illness, are likewise normed as ideals. This process takes types of humans (or the generalized human as a type) as given, not to be discovered through the experiment but only to be correlated with brain activity. Similarly, task design must assume that the specific task behaviors correspond to discrete mental "functions." It might be suspected that if results are found indicating that different brain activity is correlated with each task or group, this verifies the human or task typology. This assumes, however, that the contrary— finding no significant difference—would be meaningful. Instead, the finding of no significance is interpreted as a need for better equipment. Psychiatrist and neuroscientist Nancy Andreasen stated this very clearly in a 1997 review of the field:

> There are, at present, no known biological diagnostic markers for any mental illnesses except dementias such as Alzheimer's disease. The to-be-discovered lesions that define the remainder of mental illnesses are likely to be occurring at complex or small-scale levels that are difficult to visualize and measure" (Andreasen 1997, pp. 1586– 1587).

STAGE 2: MEASURING BRAIN ACTIVITY, FROM TRACER-MOLECULE TO CONCEPTUAL DATASET

DUMIT: I am interested in how you read images. There is a lot of literature on how radiologists read X-rays, but there isn't that much on what it means to read a PET scan. Just because it is a functional image, you seem to have to know a lot more about how this particular image was done to look at it.

TER-POGOSSIAN: I think in many instances—not in all instances, but in many instances—it is very fundamentally wrong to try and read a PET image the way you read a radiological image, because of the fact that if you read a PET image that way, well, instinctively you know that what you are looking at is not morphology but, as you said, a function. But sometimes, if you are an individual who is acquainted with x-ray pictures, you tend to think in terms of morphology, and that is a profound mistake if you do that. A hot area may represent living tissue; on the other hand, it may represent dead tissue just as well. The sooner you get away from the morphology concept, the better off you will be. You do have to relate your images to morphology; you have to know which organ you are in and which portion of the organ you are in. But beyond that . . . this is one of the reasons why there has been a divergence between radiologists and internists in nuclear medicine. Radiologists are very, very morphologically inclined. Internists are much more physiologically inclined, biochemically inclined. An internist knows the biochemistry.

A PET image, in so many ways, is not like any other image. Not only is the physiological, functional nature of the underlying data a problem conceptually for most of us, both doctors and laypersons but, also, the quantitative dataset itself is dynamic and always imperfectly represented visually. The layers of construction making up the image can literally "make it up."

The PET scanner itself is only one of the many technologies needed to gather and process the data. First, the radioactive substance has to be made. PET scanning relies on a specific type of radioactivity, positron emission, which is produced by a limited set of isotopes. These positron emitters, however, include carbon-12, oxygen-15, nitrogen-13, and fluorine-18. Carbon, oxygen, nitrogen, and hydrogen are the basic building-block atoms of life. Because fluorine can substitute for hydrogen atoms in molecules, almost any molecule of significance for studying the brain can be made radioactive and its activity can be tracked in a PET scanner. Crucially, these positron emitters have relatively short half-lives, meaning that they do not stay radioactive in the body too long (unlike carbon-14, which lasts for centuries). Table 3.2 lists the most common positron emitters.[18]

Table 3.2
Half-Lives of Positron Emitters

Radionuclide	Half-life (minutes)
Carbon-11	20.4
Nitrogen-13	10.0
Oxygen-15	2.1
Fluorine-18	110.0

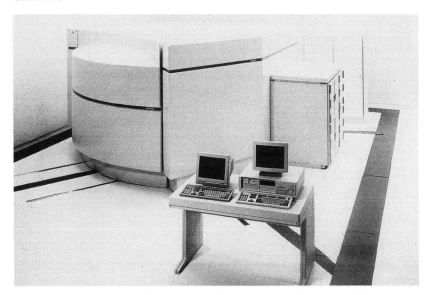

FIGURE 3.3. CTI cylcotron. (From *Technical Introduction: ECAT Scanners*; reproduced by permission of Siemens Medical Solutions USA, Inc.)

The short half-life of these isotopes is a drawback, though. It means that the isotopes must be produced on-site or very nearby. They also need to be produced in a cyclotron, which accelerates protons fast enough to cause target atoms to lose electrons and become radioactive isotopes (figure 3.3). Cyclotrons are fairly large, requiring a medium-size room shielded for radiation; are quite expensive (about $1 million to $2 million); and require expert technical assistance to run.[19] The necessity of a cyclotron is one of the factors that limit more widespread PET scanning.[20]

Once the isotope is produced, it is still not ready to be used. Because a PET scanner can theoretically trace any life molecule, a crucial decision in all PET experiments is which molecule to track. Nuclear chemists working in "hot chemistry" labs can replace atoms of regular molecules with radioisotopes, creating radiolabeled molecules. These radiotracers behave *exactly* as their nonradioactive siblings do.[21] The idea of labeling with radioisotopes goes back to Georg von Hevesy, who won a Nobel prize in 1934 for discovering the tracer principle. Henry Wagner Jr. described it to me this way:

> Do you know how the tracer principal was invented? Hevesy worked for [Ernest] Rutherford as a Ph.D. student, and he was given the project of separating radioactive lead from stable lead. That was his

thesis, to separate those two. But he found that no matter what he tried, physical or chemical, he couldn't separate them. So instead of this being a total failure, he said, "This will be a tracer of lead." Because it has exactly the same physical and chemical properties, it is impossible to separate them.

This story, part of the lore of nuclear medicine, is often repeated in books and in talks.[22] Combining the elements of a detective story with creative scientific insight, the tale functions as a symbolic reference for the nuclear medicine community's purpose.

The actual preparation of the radiotracer involves making sure of its purity, chemically combining it with other molecules to produce the radioactive target molecule, and packaging it to be used. In the case of standard molecules such as water and glucose, this process has been automated (called a black box) and is often a part of the cyclotron (figure 3.4).

Theoretically, the tracer principle allows any molecule — oxygen gas, carbon dioxide, glucose, and drugs such as Prozac and cocaine — to be labeled and its activity through physiological and chemical transformations to be followed.[23] As Phelps explained in the introduction, a radiotracer is an ideal participant observer because it behaves exactly like its nonradioactive counterpart. A more precise analog of the radiotracer is a surveillance bug that transmits the position and/or conversations of the person being bugged.

Because the tracer is what is emitting the radioactivity, an image of "brain activity" is really an image of glucose consumption, oxygen flow, Prozac flow, and so on. Debates over tracer choice are concerned with the ability of different tracers to stand in for and represent neuronal or brain activity. There are cases, for example, in which glucose consumption and oxygen flow "decouple," meaning that they do not behave the same during the same task, posing a problem for comparing results of "brain activation" across different tracers. The concept of "brain activation" is thus a problem of "chemical resolution" in which the activity of a single type of molecule is substituted for the brain processes.

The production of the radiotracer has to be coordinated temporally and spatially with the preparation of the subject to be scanned and the scanner. In the case of fluorine-18, the subject must be ready for injection and testing; in the case of oxygen or carbon, the subject must be already in the scanner. The radiotracer, once injected, flows through the body just like the regular molecule, but it emits radioactivity in the form of positrons. Positrons are positively charged electrons that travel quite randomly 1 to 7 millimeters[24] before colliding with an electron, resulting in the annihilation of both and the emission of two gamma rays shoot-

71

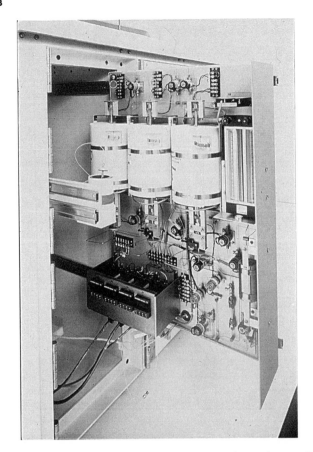

FIGURE 3.4 Automated isotope production. "Fluorodeoxyglucose (FDG) synthesis module from CTI, Inc. This particular device uses the radioisotope Flourine[18] (18-F) produced by the cyclotron and through various chemical reactions, produces sterile, chemically pure FDG. Several chemical reactions occur, and the typical synthesis takes about one hour from the delivery of the 18-F." (From *Technical Introduction: ECAT Scanners*; reproduced by permission of Siemens Medical Solutions USA, Inc.)

ing off almost 180 degrees apart. Millions of positrons are released every minute, and each release results in two gamma rays (figure 3.5).

The PET scanner itself looks like a large metal doughnut standing up, with a table running through the middle of it and wires trailing off the bottom. The early PETT III scanner had its guts visible (see figure 3.6). Because the procedure involves radioactivity, the scanner room also must be shielded. The subject lies down on the table, and his or her

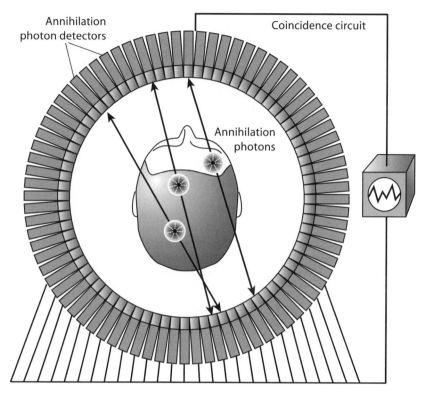

FIGURE 3.5. Coincidence detection. (Posner and Raichle 1994)

head is aligned and firmly fixed. The slightest movement of the head during the scanning process will cause artifacts in the resulting scan.[25]

The inside of the doughnut consists of hundreds of special crystals that are capable of capturing gamma rays. Gamma rays that enter a crystal have a good chance of colliding with an atom in it and releasing a photon of light. There are different crystals to choose from, each a different trade-off between stopping power, speed of multiple captures, durability, and cost. The photon of light then travels through the crystal to a "photomultiplier tube," which magnifies the light power so that it can be registered by a light detector.[26]

The crystals and light detectors are arranged in a doughnut fashion to take advantage of the fact that the gamma rays travel almost directly opposite each other. When two detectors are triggered at almost exactly the same time, as measured by a "coincidence circuit," the scanner presumes that a positron must have been emitted on or very near the line between the two crystals (see Plate 3 [steps 1 through 3]). Very fast

73

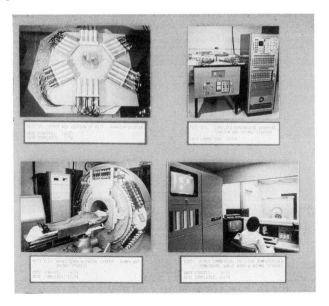

FIGURE 3.6. Four early PET scanners, called PETT (positron emission transaxial tomography). These scanners were produced at Washington University, St. Louis. (Courtesy of Michael Phelps)

crystals and electronics can also measure the microsecond difference between the two triggers and make a good guess as to where on the line the presumed positron was.

The positron is only a "presumed" positron because there are a number of factors that add noise to the data collection process. The first occurs because of the high number of positrons released: Two positrons may result in two pairs of gamma rays striking crystals at about the same time, causing false coincidences to be detected.

Gamma rays can also be deflected or absorbed while still in the head, causing missed or misaligned coincidences. Finally, a gamma ray can pass through a crystal into the adjacent one. In each case, there is no possible way to know that a coincidence is false. But the high number of actual coincidences from most regions is usually enough to assume that these spurious ones can be treated as reducible noise. The net result is that the radioactivity that hits the doughnut is assumed to be the result of radiotracer emission locations on the lines between the crystals.[27]

Spatially, the doughnut shape of the scanner collects its data in the form of "slices" of the brain (Figure 3.7). Like bread slices, these brain slices have a thickness, here due to the thickness of the crystals. *Thick-*

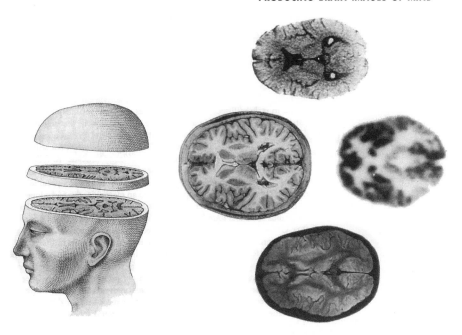

FIGURE 3.7. Brain slices. The four images at the right were generated using different techniques for imaging the brain. Starting at 9 o'clock and moving clockwise, the four techniques are standard photography, x-ray computed tomography (CT), positron emission tomography, and magnetic resonance imaging. Note first that each technique makes different structures visible, and then note second that the slice itself has a necessary thickness that each technique flattens (erases or averages) in different ways. (Posner and Raichle 1994)

ness means that the emission activity in the slice is lumped together. Smaller crystals can reduce the slice thickness but would collect fewer counts, making noise a bigger concern.

The angle of the head in the scanner introduces another aspect of the brain slice: At different angles, different brain structures lie together on the same slice (figures 3.8, a and b). The kind of angle used differs by lab because labs use different reference brain atlases to locate and correlate physical structures with the imaged ones. There is no ideal angle or atlas, but the different standards are one of the things that makes reading another lab's scans so difficult.

The choice of where to start and stop the angled slices introduces an anatomical cutoff as well. In figure 3.8b, the slices end above the bulblike cerebellum at the bottom of the brain. Nancy Andreasen has observed that this kind of choice builds in key assumptions about which regions of the brain *could* be involved in the activity:

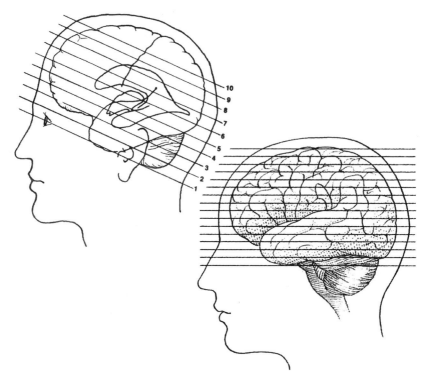

FIGURE 3.8. Brain slice angles. These images were taken from two different books on brain imaging. They represent competing standard ways of slicing the brain. The different angles create differently shaped images, and on those images different brain structures appear together. (Images drawn from Andreason 1984 and from Posner and Raichle 1994)

Although early PET studies simply cut off the cerebellum, based on the assumption that it could not be doing anything of interest to students of cognition and emotion, more recent studies have indicated that it is used in many different kinds of mental activity . . . (Andreasen 2001, p. 72)

Also, because of the angles within which the crystals collect the gamma rays, the slices are not, in fact, uniformly thick the way that bread slices are; they are bulged in the middle. Said a senior PET researcher:

You don't think of a slice that is infinitely thin, the way, say, a physicist would approach it, or a thermodynamicist would say it has no meaning until you go to an infinitely thin slice. No, I'm always interested in the fact that if I've got a one-centimeter cube, first of all, what is the function of that cube? And then, what is the biochemistry going on in that cube, and why?

Finally, the architecture of the scanner affects the form of data gathered in each brain slice. Each different scanner shape — thin ring, thick doughnut, hexagonal, fixed, or rotating — is better at detecting some areas than others. For instance, some scanners collect better data from the center of the brain, with the periphery having more noise, whereas other scanners have the opposite trade-off. Each of these different spatial collection issues is still being studied by PET researchers. Each contributes to the concept of the "brain slice activity" as a representation of the collected coincidence counts.

A difficulty often noted by researchers is the extreme differences of appearances of PET images from different institutions. C. L. Grady examined the differences in data produced by two different machines and discovered that even for the same person, "there was no simple interaction between the complex structure of the brain and differences in performance characteristics of the two tomographs" (Grady 1991). This finding illustrates the problem with PET being uniquely able to measure brain molecular flow rates at this level of resolution. Because it provides information unobtainable from other measures, there is no way at present to confirm the results. "If [such a large] difference . . . can be obtained on the same subjects with the same injection using different tomographs, then apparent differences in metabolic rates reported by different groups should be interpreted with caution" (Grady 1991).

The next conceptual dimension of data collection is time. Scanning takes time: 2 minutes for oxygen scans and 30 minutes for FDG, for example. Radioactivity rates decrease by half each half-life, so activity during the latter part of a scan must be modified to account for this fact. In addition, the process being measured, brain activity, is dynamically changing during this period. Thus the data being collected consist of a "slice of time" that is necessarily lumped together into a "state of activation."[28]

At this point, then, data has been collected on millions of coincidence lines in conceptual brain slices over a period of time. All this data is collected into a computer, and the lines are mathematically "reconstructed" into a slice-shaped dataset of emission data, a graphically organized array of numbers. As in the rest of PET research, there are a number of competing approaches, in this case to the algorithms used to solve the problem of the most likely dataset that could have resulted in the actual data received (see Plate 3 [steps 4 through 9]). The result is a grid of activity in which each box in the grid represents numerically the reconstructed amount of activity for a small section (or *voxel*) of the brain slice over the period of the scan.

This division of the brain slice into voxels creates a new concept: a *functional brain region* that is given to represent the average amount of brain activation in that box of the brain over the period of time of the scan.[29] For any voxel, the accuracy of the count number is subject to what is called the partial volume effect, however, which is the spillover into a voxel from adjacent voxels that have significantly higher radioactivity, resulting in a number of voxels that will be represented as having more activity than they should have. A related issue is the overlooking of regions of high radioactivity that are much smaller than the voxel size. Here the voxel will be registered at a lower average rate, and the area of high activity will be missed.

This uniqueness is also a problem for researchers with the newest and best-resolution tomographs who report activation in structures no other institution can even measure (see Plate 11). The physical theory of PET concludes that only structures larger than twice the size of the resolution, or "full width at half maximum (FWHM)" can be properly measured. Structures smaller than this are so affected by surrounding areas that they cannot be reliably interpreted (Karp et al. 1991; Mazziotta and Phelps 1985).

> Once an image is obtained, the procedure to extract regional values will also affect the regional quantitation. The most common procedure is to delineate an anatomical area into the PET scan images and then obtain its average value. The size and geometry of the region of interest [ROI] will affect the quantitative values obtained. Size is important because in order to obtain adequate quantitation the dimensions of the ROI should be at least twice the spatial resolution of the system. In brain studies attempting to quantify gray matter activity, this will introduce a source of error because the mean width of the cortex is 3 mm. Cortical regions will include activity from surrounding areas. (Volkow et al. 1991, p. 133)

Each increase in resolution reveals a whole new world of structures. One kind of ideal PET machine would have a resolution small enough to show each neuron, but no one knows what these pictures would even begin to look like.

Brain slice thickness and reconstruction of the slice into voxels determine what is called the "spatial resolution" of the PET scanner, defined as the voxel size. Spatial resolution directly determines what scale of brain activity is detected and represented and what scales are ignored.

In a similar manner, the time resolution of the device determines activity that registers consistently over the time-slice of data collection and ignores shorter-in-time peaks and valleys of activity in voxels as well as longer changes that happen to overlap with the specific time slice chosen. The net result is the concepts of a "functional brain region," "activation," and a "functional map of the brain's activity" that are always produced by the PET apparatus.[30] Functional brain regions do not exist in the brain where neurons are in constant cross-talk with each other using a variety of electrical, chemical, and physiological means at spatial scales of nanometers and time scales of nanoseconds. Instead, the PET apparatus produces the functional brain region as a discrete, measurable, locatable, and ideally nameable time-space voxel of the brain that can be correlated with the person's state or trait.

To recap, the steps in creating a brainset are as follows:

1. A one-to-one mapping of a data set of quantities onto a three-dimensional voxelized model of the brain is done.
2. The dataset is the result of a simulation of flow rates of the radiopharmaceutical in the brain.
3. The flowrates are reconstructed by a mathematical algorithm on the decay counts.
4. The decay counts are statistical indicators of the spatial and temporal distribution of the radiopharmaceutical.
5. The radiopharmaceutical is presumably tracing a significant biological process.
6. The biological process is hoped to be significantly related to brain activity, which in turn, is hoped to be related to cognitive and behavioral tasks.

These six relationships are *each* treated as the referent of PET images in different scientific articles, depending, for instance, on whether the authors are involved in chemically producing the tracer, calculating the flow rate, or providing the task.

All of these processes of data collection have been continually critiqued and revised since the 1980s. Each revision of scanner and reconstruction software often involves trade-offs between sensitivity or efficiency, spatial resolution, and speed. Each of these trade-offs emphasizes a different aspect of the radiotracer activity being measured, which then has implications for the assessment of the brain activity being measured. For instance, with greater spatial resolution, researchers might be able to image smaller brain areas, thus producing more detailed maps of functional circuits. With greater sensitivity, however, tinier amounts of radioactivity are needed to make accurate images, allowing either greater differentiation of levels of activity in different regions or greater time resolution, images of shorter duration that possibly emphasize different kinds of brain processes.

These debates hint at the tremendous difficulty of addressing the brain as a whole through the measurement of a tiny subset of its parts. At the same time, it is precisely through such assertion of measures and the reasoned critiques of them that new notions and measures of brain activity are invented (Danziger 1990b). In the end, the ideal for the rest of the experiment is that the whole of stage 2 is standardized, or at least black-boxed in the absence of settling it.

In sum, in stage 2, measuring a brain entails reconstructing it as a dataset. The process of brain imaging always ends with this result: that the brain is knowable as a set of combinatorial states. According to media philosopher Vilém Flusser, this mode of knowing/perceiving begins with the photograph. Both PET and the photographic apparatus can be understood as containing an incredibly large yet finite set of possible products: pictures viewed as different combinations of colored or grayscale dots. The number of combinations may not be imaginable, but it is not infinite. Flusser's insight is that an apparatus like this defines a combinatorial space that is conceptual: The picture's dots express the concepts of grayscale, a pixellated discrete world, and a combinatorial universe (Flusser 1984).

With regard to brain imaging, and PET scanning in particular, understanding the apparatus in Flusser's manner allows us to identify the concepts that replace the biological brain in the images: The dataset is discrete, volumetric, and timeless. Despite early attempts to make brain imaging into movies (Wagner, etc.), the movies were too hard to read. The images are discrete in that a quantitative amount of hits is understood as a "level of activity" represented by a single number. This number is defined by a three-dimensional location in the space of the skull, and the location of the number is a voxel, a three-dimensional box (Beaulieu 2000).

Different scanner architectures, crystal counting techniques, and correction algorithms result in different datasets on the "same" brain. There is no ideal scanner or isotope because the brain does not have voxels or levels of activities or discrete events. The overall conceptual object produced by the apparatus of the PET scanner is a three-dimensional space filled with discrete, adjacent boxes, each containing a single number for each state in time. This conceptual object takes the place of the brain in subsequent stages. We note, though, that the final conceptual object, the *brainset*, is analogous to the cognitive neuroscience assumption that the brain itself is analyzable into separate module-like components that are differentially active in a state-like manner. The

PET apparatus builds these neuroscience assumptions into its architecture and thus can *appear* to confirm them, while necessarily reinforcing them.

STAGE 3: MAKING DATA COMPARABLE

> Using methods called "image processing" . . . the computer acts as an extension of the eye and the brain by selecting information the scientists cannot see. (Blumenthal 1982)

The scanner has now produced a brainset, an apparently stable set of numbers that represent the flow rate of the tracer and apparent activation. The next stage of the process of producing a brain image consists in first adjusting and transforming the dataset so that it corresponds to some other brainset, either the subject's own MRI, for instance, or a reference brainset. In the first case, the PET data is computationally combined, or "registered," with the MRI information so that the activity voxels can be given anatomical locations. Often this is combined with the process of then transforming or warping the subject's brainset into a standardized human brainset or "atlas." As Anne Beaulieu describes in "The Space Inside the Skull," this process presumes the meaningful and practical possibility of a *generalized human brain*, and then produces it (Beaulieu 2000).

The following discussion of different brain atlases by MRI imager Matthew Brett, illustrates some of the difficulties:

> The MNI [Montréal Neurological Institute] defined a new standard brain by using a large series of MRI scans on normal controls. Recall that the Talairach brain is the brain dissected and photographed for the famous Talairach and Tournoux atlas. The atlas has Brodmann's [anatomical] areas labelled, albeit in a rather approximate way. In fact, what the authors did was to look at pictures of the Brodmann map and estimate where the same place was on their brain. To quote from the atlas, p. 10: "The brain presented here was not subjected to histological studies and the transfer of the cartography of Brodmann usually pictured in two-dimensional projections sometimes possesses uncertainties."
>
> The MNI wanted to define a brain that is more representative of the population. They therefore did a large number of MRI scans on normal subjects [305 of them], and did a simple linear match of each brain to the brain in the Talairach atlas. . . . The problem introduced by the MNI standard brains is that the MNI linear transform has not matched the brains completely to the Talairach brain. As a result, the

MNI brains are slightly larger (in particular higher, deeper and longer) than the Talairach brain. The differences are larger as you get further from the middle of the brain, towards the outside, and are at maximum in the order of 10mm. (Brett 1999)[31]

There are many techniques for transforming and mapping the three-dimensional PET and MRI data onto each other. Various warping techniques include (1) finding standard landmarks and "stretching" the dataset[32]; (2) registering the data to the subject's magnetic resonance image and then transforming the image to match the atlas, (3) warping on the basis of the surface of the brain, and (4) performing a nonlinear three-dimensional warping of brain structures. Each of these methods, of course, has trade-offs, and is still being debated and adjusted. The resulting compound image (MRI + PET) combines high-resolution anatomical information with quantitative physiological data.[33] Each of these methods trades off precision in one realm for accuracy in another.

The net result is that all the brainsets are rendered comparable to each other and each activity voxel can be located within the atlas and given a more or less precise anatomical location (e.g., in the basal ganglia). Unfortunately, there is disagreement between many labs over the proper reference brain—the Talairach atlas, for instance, was generated from a woman in her sixties who died shortly after having an MRI. Consequently, brain data located on one atlas is not easily comparable with other atlases without significant work (Beaulieu 2000; Talairach 1957; Talairach and Tournoux 1988).

Brainsets often must be normalized to each other in activity levels. In some people, the overall flow in each hemisphere is slightly different. To assist in comparing regions between the two hemispheres, they are often adjusted so that they are of the same average overall activity. Then, because voxel activity measures are dependent on total isotope emission activity, people with higher metabolisms will tend to have higher overall brain blood flow. Because most labs are interested in regional activity, the relative difference in activity in one voxel compared with another, the total overall amount of voxel activity is usually adjusted so that comparisons can be made across individuals. In this case, the absolute activity is defined as not relevant to the study.[34]

Once the brainsets are made into comparable brainsets, the work of extracting significance from them can begin. Significance in PET brain imaging is usually defined as regional differences in activation between two brainsets—for example, the set of voxels corresponding to the basal ganglia are more active in this brainset of an anxious person than in the brainset of the same person when calm. As discussed earlier, these differences can be between the brainsets of an individual doing one task and the same individual doing another one, between two individuals doing the same task, between an individual with a condition (like schizophrenia) and one without, or between two groups of individuals.

In each case, the emphasis is on determining which voxels of activity differ enough between the two brainsets to suggest that the anatomical location of these voxels—a specific brain region—is "involved" in whatever defines the comparison. For example, brainsets of an individual looking at a colored pattern compared with brainsets of the same individual looking at the same pattern in black and white reveal that a set of voxels identified as located in part of the visual cortex had 10 percent more activity. The suggestion of this data is that part of the visual cortex is "correlated with seeing color" or with "color processing." Because all that can be determined is correlation, this kind of study cannot prove that the brain region is involved or responsible for the function of color processing. Instead, PET scanning is often described as "hypothesis-generating" (suggesting brain regions that might be involved in an activity) rather than "hypothesis-confirming."

This example also demonstrates that PET must conceptually assume that activation change is significant and represents the "participation" of the "area" (set of voxels) differentially activated in the correlated task. Activation is also conceptual, understood as linear: More is better—more activation means more participation in the function. The corollary of this assumption is that voxels that do not differ between two brainsets are not involved in the task or comparison. In the living brain, all areas are "constantly" active, except the areas that are dead due to, for example, stroke. All of the neurons are in use, oxygen and glucose are being consumed, and neurotransmitters are being released and taken in.

When images are colored (discussed later) only the voxels that differ are given colors, and the other voxels are often rendered black. Comments made to the effect that "no other areas were active" point to the visual and conceptual acceptance of the brainset as the brain. These are shorthand phrases that fill in for "were differentially more active," but they act to reinforce the notion that the other areas of the brain *could* be uninvolved, because they were "off."

Methods of comparing images and determining significance vary from lab to lab. (It may seem tedious to repeat yet another reminder of process differences between labs, but there is no other way to demonstrate the complexity of the interacting layers of assumptions underlying a PET image and how each of these assumptions is not standard within the PET field but contested.) The example just described involved *subtraction*. The value of each voxel in the black-and-white brainset was subtracted from the corresponding voxel in the color brainset. Ideally, most corresponding voxels will have been equal in value, subtracting to zero, implying that the brain activity in that voxel was not affected by the difference between the tasks. The resulting brainset thus highlights those voxels that differed (see Plate 4, top row).

Conceptually, subtracting one image from another assumes that regions of the brain that show no overall change in activity are not directly involved in the task or condition. This is an assumption similar to that with a computer's hardware, where the math coprocessor heats up only when algorithms needing certain functions are run. However, in computers without a math coprocessor, the same functions can be programmed into regular RAM (random-access memory). In this case, there is no overall difference in any particular component when the computer performs the algorithms. The RAM is critically involved in and directly responsible for those functions, but it is also involved in database manipulations and Internet surfing at the same intensity. Consequently, an "image" of the latter computer would not detect the role of the RAM program in performing the algorithms because the functional difference is "hidden" as a difference in coding within a constant-use unit, not "present" in a specific, dedicated unit.

A second analogy will further constrain this concept of activation. Assume that we want to detect the top tennis players in a country but are able to measure only general muscle intensity of its inhabitants. We might try to correlate the intensity of activity with tennis tournaments and hypothesize that the top tennis players will be more active during tournaments than not. But what if these tennis professionals also spend every day practicing at great intensity? Then even if they do the work of playing tennis for the country, they will not be detectable through correlation with tennis events. Analogously, we might wonder about regions of the brain that "practice" analyzing patterns of color during the time that they are not actually analyzing new color input.

A different paradigm that competes with the concept of participative activation is that of individual differences and learning. Richard Haier, for instance, designed a study of people playing the computer game Tetris in which scans were done of people (1) just learning to play, (2) as they were becoming more skilled, and (3) when they could play the game consistently at its highest level. Correlating these images, he claims to have found that some specific regions of the brain were more active when learning, then got less active as the person became more skilled, and finally were less active than at rest when the person was playing as an expert. He described this data as conforming to an "efficiency hypothesis," in which a brain region is very active when adapting to a new task and then over time the region becomes very streamlined or efficient at that task and therefore needs less and less activity to carry it out. In the final instance, one can imagine the region on a kind of autopilot, less active even than when it is not performing the activity at all (and perhaps participating obliquely in other tasks).

The efficiency hypothesis is useful to highlight the particular design of most cognitive science tasks. They are specifically chosen as those kinds of tasks that people do not tend to get better at. Thus, they are suited to repeating over and over with the same person and—it is hoped—to causing the same response behaviorally and neurologically each time. Equally, they allow many different people to be tested without worrying about how good they are at the task. The functional brain map of cognitive neuroscience tends to be a map of those functions for which there is little or no learning. This abstraction of the range of human functions is common to much of psychology today and has captured much of PET scanner research.

Having clarified the paradigms of isolation of tasks in brainsets of individuals through subtraction, we can now attend to how these results can be combined with each other to produce results in groups. The basic method is one of averaging (see Plate 4, middle and bottom rows). In the case of the color-seeing task, the subtracted brainsets of each of five individuals are normalized to each other as described: Their average activity level is altered to the same average, and the brainsets are deformed to the same absolute reference brain atlas. Now the same voxel value in each normalized brainset can be added together and divided by the total number of brainsets to provide the average group voxel value. Repeating for each voxel, the end result is a new "average group brainset."

This average brainset is intriguing because it has conceptualized significant activity as only the subtracted activity that is most common to the set of individual brainsets. Subtracted activity that is common to only one or two is redefined from being potential "individual participative activity" to "noise." This individual variability is often not represented at all in the resultant average brainset, being rendered black. This is intentional. Individual differences are treated as noise in cognitive psychology, whose mission is to discover the baseline mental functions that are common to (most) normal people. What is retained as significant in the averaged brainsets are those regions that can be said to participate in the task in most individuals.

The study of patients, to investigate the recovery of language functions, raises further problems, in particular whether it is appropriate to average patient data. The answer in many cases is likely to be that it is inappropriate . . . mixing the results from patients reveals only common features, and individual differences of great potential interest are obscured. However, the comparison of an individual patient's results with grouped normal data, to look for significant regional differences, is a relatively insensitive technique, and one that is open to problems of interpretation — for example, does the patient show a regional difference from normal subjects because of an adaptive change in the neural networks processing the task, or because of an irrelevant stimulus such as discomfort from a full bladder of which the investigator was unaware at the time the patient was studied? Irrelevant stimuli are likely to be randomly distributed amongst a group of normal subjects, and therefore conveniently "lost" during inter-subject averaging. (Wise et al. 1991)

Turning back now to the example figure (Plate 4), another conceptual abstraction can be discovered. The five subtracted brainsets each have a fairly lateralized activation in the visual cortex, meaning that the left side is significantly more active than the corresponding right side, or vice versa. The average brainset, however, is prominently bilateral, with both the left and right side of the visual cortex showing high (white) subtracted activity. Thus, the process of averaging here produces a new *quality* in the average brainset that is not present in any of its source brainsets. When I have discussed this image with other brain-imaging researchers, the most common response has been, "Yes, that is right, but if you think that is bad, let me tell you a story . . ." The point of their stories is that there are many such inherent but well-known risks in every algorithm. The key is keeping them from ending up in the results section of the journal article, not in keeping them out of the images (see below under "Extreme Images").

Averaging can be also be done before subtracting images. A group of brainsets of schizophrenic patients might be averaged together, and then an averaged brainset from a group of normal controls can be subtracted from it. In this case, the difference between the normal subjects' brainsets and the differences between the schizophrenic subjects' brainsets are filtered out as noise first, and only the group-shared intensities are subtracted. This result is then interpreted as potentially specific to "schizophrenic brains."

This is a two-step process. First, the selected (super)schizophrenic patients are scanned and their brainsets averaged, creating an "average schizophrenic subjects–group brainset." Already, the presumption to be able to meaningfully average together a group of schizophrenic subjects is sliding into the notion of a "schizophrenic brainset." This is to be compared with the "average (super)normals-group brainset," interpreted as a "normal brainset." In the second step, the normal brainset is subtracted from the schizophrenic brainset, with the result suggesting a "brainset of schizophrenia itself"—that is, the disease is presented as the "only" difference between the two groups, all other difference, it is hoped, having been eliminated as noise.

Difference between brain images is another one of the words, such as *significance*, whose multiple meanings often ambiguously and productively play off of each other. Here the difference (as nonsimilarity) between the two groups is layered on top of the difference (as the result of an arithmetic subtraction) between the two brainsets.

Identifying areas of the averaged brainset that are significant is the province of computational algorithm writers who debate the relative merits of each system.

PETER FOX: I started playing around with the first spatial normalization routines, with Talairach and figuring out how to use skull landmarks as ways to normalize, and developed a scheme of it that I could do with a ruler and a calculator. I presented it at a lab meeting, and everybody like it. So Joel [Perlmutter] said that he would be willing to code it. He did, and everybody used it. It was the laboratory standard.

[In terms of] developing the averaging, [Mark] Mintun and [Eric M.] Reiman and myself talked about it a lot. Then we began kind of arguing out the steps, because averaging sounds easy, but there are a lot of steps involved. You have to mask the data, and there are a lot of interim steps. So we would argue through the steps, then code it, then test it. We kept playing with it—the automatic search routine, the local maxima searching—so when you have this big cluster of pixels that you can talk about it in some more precise way. That algorithm developed by sitting and fooling around with a region and kind of floating a region around in 2-D to see how reproducible it was to find a center of mass based on a moving region. It turned out that it was reproducible, and I sat down and figured out how to do it in a third dimension, again with paper and pencil, and then took that to Mintun. I said, "I can reduce these to a three-dimensional center of mass between slices," and I had the data. I collected the data and showed him how reproducible it was between subjects. So he then did some computer simulations and tested the robustness of it, and demonstrated really elegantly how precisely that could be done. Then again, that was more software that we then applied to the data.

We went and talked to statisticians on and off and found them generally struggling with the problem and not understanding. . . . It was so different from anything that they had done that they didn't have much to say. So ultimately, with a lot of the statistics—

87

and the same is true for [Karl] Friston and the SPM [statistical parametric mapping]—it was developed by the people who wanted to use it, and then it was critiqued by the statisticians. If you go to them—again, fairly universal experience—you go to a statistician and say we have this problem, our data structure is like this and our question is this, they'll say: "Wow, that is a hard problem." You say, "I know. What is the solution?" They say, "I don't know." If you [could have caught] their interest, maybe they could have solved it.

But really what happened is that people got out statistics textbooks and started reading and started learning about probability theory and the central-limit theorem and began trying to see how to apply those principles to our datasets. Friston wasn't a statistician. Friston is a psychiatrist, but . . .

Dumit: He had a problem to solve . . .

Fox: He had a problem to solve—that is exactly right. And got deeper and deeper into the statistical theory and coded all of that himself. I mean, all of that SPM stuff, Friston personally coded. He learned how to use MATLAB [software for data analysis], and he generated it all.

There are different assumptions built into each kind of statistical algorithm. Most algorithms *always* highlight one or more brain regions— they choose the *highest* peaks, for example. As such, they cannot be used to disconfirm the premise that there are active brain regions (Uttal 2001, p. 185). The fundamental point of contention between different approaches is that there is no other method of proving what significant brain activation should look like. Should a set of voxels be interpreted via a center-of-mass algorithm as Fox described or using SPM as Friston uses or via a field activation approach as Per Roland argues in *Brain Activation*? (Roland 1993). At the present time, these are all competing approaches to analyzing brainset data for significance.

Finally, data on individuals from different machines and different institutions can be combined into a large database of "human brain anatomy and function." The Institute of Medicine set up a National Neural Circuitry Database Committee in October 1989 to evaluate how such a database might be constructed. This committee's difficulty with levels of analysis of brain data led to the publication of a set of priorities and recommendations for pilot studies, *Mapping the Brain and Its Functions: Integrating Enabling Technologies into Neuroscience Research* (Pechura and Martin 1991), a book which features four PET scans on its cover (see Plate 14). The Human Brain Project is another project funded as a result of this effort, and it includes grants for BrainMap and the Probabilistic Atlas (National Institutes of Health 1993). BrainMap is a distributed computer program (distributed across several physical locations and connected through the Internet) that integrates information from peer-reviewed studies of the functional brain so they may be cross-referenced by anatomical location (Beaulieu 2000; Fox and Woldorff 1994). The Probabilistic Atlas is an attempt to correlate scales of information about the brains of normal subjects matched for handedness, age, and gender with variability across different populations (Mazziotta et al. 1995).[35]

These techniques of averaging, subtracting, and databasing are both very powerful and very tricky in terms of evaluation and significance. These techniques emphasize similarities across individuals and treat differences between them as "noise" (irrelevant information). They necessarily presume that there is no significant anatomical variability in the functions being studied (Fox and Pardo 1991). These techniques have been successfully and prominently used in the study of language, for instance, in spite of studies that have shown widespread individual variability:

> Mapping of cortical language sites by stimulation studies of the surgically exposed dominant hemisphere demonstrates that there is tremendous inter-individual variability in the location of essential language areas. . . . Many of these areas fall outside the classically delineated Wernicke's and Broca's areas. Furthermore, any specific zone within Wernicke's or Broca's area was found to be essential for language in less than half of the cases. . . . It is apparent that the variability of language organization is so great that a mapping procedure must be carried out in each individual for whom language localization is important. (Martin et al. 1990, citing Ojemann 1979 and Ojemann et al. 1989)

The issue of variability is not unaddressed within most PET articles, but it is subordinated to PET's ability to generate statistically significant results. Calling attention to this subordination, one editorial was entitled, "Can Statistics Cause Brain Damage?" (Ford 1983). This is not the place to examine critiques of PET statistics but to simply acknowledge that these issues are undergoing lively debate within the corridors, discussions, and appendixes, of the PET community.[36] The most significant conceptual concern seems to be whether, and where, PET should be used as inferential (hypothesis-confirming) or exploratory (hypothesis-generating). Rapoport reports on the "heated" discussion of this issue at a 1989 workshop on PET data analysis, relating to "whether it is better to avoid type I errors (where a statistically significant positive finding proves erroneous) rather than type II errors (where statements of statistical insignificance prove erroneous)" (Rapoport 1991, p. A142).[37] Rapoport appeared to lean toward the exploratory use of PET, where results are presented that may be wrong but that can spark further studies.

STAGE 4: PRODUCING INTERPRETED IMAGES

> Inferences drawn from qualitative in vivo measurements . . . must be viewed with extreme caution despite their intuitive visual appeal. Unfortunately, this sort of inference is the rule rather than the exception.
> (Perlmutter and Raichle 1986).

> Parenthetically, the [PET scan] pictures that are particularly attractive that you have seen in general are fairly heavily doctored, in the sense of making them more attractive than they should be.
> —Michel M. Ter-Pogossian

Significant, correlated difference, having been determined in the form of voxels, now must be made visible. This dataset of quantitative results can now be mapped onto a spatial coordinate system and displayed on a computer screen as a brainset (Wolf 1981a). Although the resulting image is two-dimensional, the brainset is actually three-dimensional, where the third dimension is typically represented using color or brightness (see Plate 9).

Peter Galison describes a historical process in which mechanical objectivity—the insistence on the natural transfer of the real objects to image—gives way to an improved object: the interpreted image (Galison 1997, p. 349). The interpreted image is seen as a more "realistic" process because it can be recognized by nonspecialists. "For the image to be purely 'natural' was for it to become, *ipso facto*, as obscure as the nature it was supposed to depict" (p. 351).

DUMIT: One of the strengths of PET is that it gives you quantitative data. And at the same time you produce visual, qualitative images. How do these two things work together? Can you read images?

WAGNER: There is a tremendous amount of data. When you say *quantification*, you are talking about numbers, and these spatially oriented studies, these four-dimensional studies, three dimensions in space and one dimension in time, can only be abstracted and displayed in a meaningful way in the form of images. Otherwise there are too many numbers. Your brain can't really handle more than a couple of variables at one time if they are quantitative, so you have to have abstractions. And images are a very, very nice way of abstracting quantification.

Starting with the normalized brainset or with the averaged subtracted brainset, the primary problem is how to make sure the reader can understand both the location of the voxels of significance and the meaning of the (relative) activity values. The "simplest" method is to assign each number a shade of gray, starting with black for 0 and ending with white for 100, assuming that the values range from 0 to 100. Because it is not always possible or desirable, however, to present 100 shades of grayscale, decisions have to be made as to how to group different values together into different shades. This process of grouping is called "windowing," meaning that one range of values (e.g., 0–10) will be assigned to black, another range (11–20) to dark gray, and so on (figure 3.9a). If most of the variation between two images takes place between 40 and 50, however, this will render the two images nearly identical. In this case, the windows can be adjusted so that perhaps 1–35 = black, 35–40 = darkest gray, and most of the variation in color takes place along the bands 41–42, 43–44, 45–46, 47–48, and 49–50, with 50–55 being lightest gray and 56–100 being white (figure 3.9b). This windowing scheme makes the difference between the two images stand out clearly, and conceptually it makes the close similarity of the two brainsets appear not to be very similar at all. Similar to the way that voxels define a specific scale of spatial resolution and invent brain regions, here the different windows define *activity resolution* and invent a set of discrete *activation levels*, visually eliminating the variability with the levels. Voxels have become *pixels*.

A more elegant solution to the windowing problem is to use colors rather than grayscale. The use of color scales to display differences in intensities in brain images was pioneered by Louis Sokoloff at the National Institutes of Health (NIH). He explained that in digital autoradiography (one of the precursors of PET), the researcher's eye could not see all the shades of gray that could be displayed (Sokoloff 1986; Sokoloff et al. 1977). Color was introduced to make subtle distinctions visible. This consists of assigning to each subrange of numbers (the full range of which varies from, say, 1 to 100) a specific color (e.g., 1–10 = black, 11–40 = blue, 41–60 = green, 61–70 = red, 71–100 = yellow). Now the brainset can be presented as a picture, either three-dimensionally or by slice. The coloring process is very important, as the final images look very different depending on how they are colored, even if they are based on exactly the same brainset. The data is thus dynamic even after all of the transformations have been accounted for.

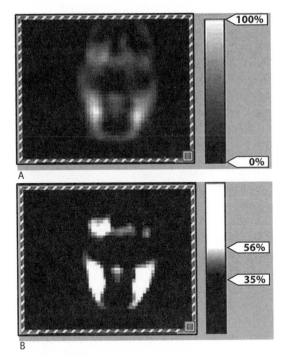

FIGURE 3.9. Gray scale differences. Figures (a) and (b) have the same numerical data set behind them, but they are colored according to two different tables of black, gray, and white rules. (Screen capture of the Image Viewer applet (ePET) developed by Val Stambolstian, Ph.D., reproduced courtesy of the Interactive Media Group, Crump Institute for Molecular Imaging)

One effect of colorizing is that new areas appear as discrete and sharply bounded, rather than diffuse.[38]

The effect can be profound. Color is not a simple linear or even two-dimensional array of values. It is best represented by some form of three-dimensional model. Choosing a set of colors to represent linear activity values is therefore an arbitrary choice. Because these colors do not correspond to the real colors of the brain, they are known as pseudo-colors. Michel Ter-Pogossian explained it this way in an interview:

> Pseudo-color exaggerates and may distort the information that is in the imaged data. There are a number of color scales, like the heated-object color scale or color mapping that the visual system knows enough about the relation of different colors to each other to be able to say, "Well, that color represents a hotter object than the other

colors." So you can order the colors. Whereas how do you order a pseudo-colored object? You can't—you can't tell whether blue is more or less than green. It is a two-dimensional color space anyway, and how you wander around in that color space is not well defined.

As with other aspects of PET, different labs have different preferred color schemes. The ePET applet is revealing in this because in addition to descriptive names for various color schemes such as "Black on White," "Hot Metal," and "Rainbow 1," there is also a location name "UCLA" (see Plate 8).

The debates over various color schemes concern clarity versus a notion of fidelity. Many color schemes, such as the rainbow one, shift from bright to dark to bright again while changing colors. This can create a significant visual shift, rendering a small change in numerical value as a solid boundary between what now appears to be two distinct regions. In this case, the spatialized brain regions of the brainset combine with the activity resolution of the windowing to create a visible "functional anatomy," regions defined as contiguous voxels all having the same color of activity. The arbitrariness of the colors reinforce the sense that these regions are internally coherent, separate from their neighbors, and therefore able to adequately represent the "functioning of the task" in question.

It must be emphasized that the criticism here is part of the aporia of visual representation of data: To make the activity visible in itself to readers, and not simply a representation of activity in general (the way that electroencephalograms often appear), there is a necessary addition of supplementary meaning. PET researchers readily describe their struggles with this problem.

DUMIT: One of the things that I am interested in is the color pictures in terms of the different things that they can signify. In one case, they can signify that there is a lot of activity going on here.

TER-POGOSSIAN: Well, yes, they signify whatever you want them to signify. This is the pitfall, of course. You can emphasize, for example, a given phenomenon very artificially, if you want to do it with color. It is misleading, too. You have to be very careful when you are using it.

DUMIT: Now when there is purple, that is going outside of the boundaries of the person's head there. Is there any significance to the mottle that is going on?

TER-POGOSSIAN: No, this is noise. That purple, that is noise; this is reconstruction noise. The reason why you see lines is that they are really reconstruction artifacts. And you see that in any reconstruction scheme, including CT scanning. However, very often you erase

93

that by just windowing it out. In other words, these represent very low values, as seen on this scale. So all you have to do is put a cutoff limit and it is removed. But that is what it is. And this, you see, this is a reconstruction artifact. Parenthetically, the pictures that are particularly attractive that you have seen in general are fairly heavily doctored, in the sense of making them more attractive than they should be.

So to answer your question, no, to the best of my knowledge there is no standardized scale. People have a tendency, of course, to use the scales that emphasize what they like to emphasize.

DUMIT: Yes, I have been struck that each different institution's pictures tend to look very different from each other. It seems very difficult to compare PET scans from different institutions.

TER-POGOSSIAN: It is very difficult. It is very, very difficult indeed. It is misleading to just use purely aesthetic values.

Ter-Pogossian here describes one of the more surprising aspects of the brainset. Despite having fixed numbers for each pixel, the ability to choose a coloring and windowing scheme allows one to use them to "signify whatever you want them to signify." The brainset is thus highly dynamic — so dynamic, in fact, that Brian Murphy, the director of computing and the PET clinical physicist in the Department of Nuclear Medicine at the State University of New York, at Buffalo produced the visually stunning set of images in Plate 12 as a cautionary visual explanation for PET physicians.

What's the difference between the 40 images [in Plate 12]? Which is normal, which has a tumor, and which has indications of stroke? Actually they're all the same image of a healthy normal volunteer — just displayed with different color scales. The effects created by various color scales may be visually dramatic but may also cause one to see distinct boundaries where there are none. With so much image analysis occurring on the computer, where dialing up any color scale you like is relatively easy, it is possible to make almost any feature stand out with the right tweaking (affectionately referred to as "dialing a defect"). For this reason, it is important to include a color scale legend somewhere on these images if they're going to be shared with others so that viewers will have some idea of how the underlying image intensity is being represented (1st and last image are presented with a linear ramp gray scale).

Note: The full series of images below appeared on the December 1996 cover of the *Journal of Nuclear Medicine Technology*. One of the motivations for creating these images (aside from their artistic merit) was to illustrate that different "interpretations" are possible for the same image under the simple artificial manipulation wrought by adjusting the color scale. An additional potential source of interpretation error was added at the time of publication—image orientation. One must be extremely careful when viewing images in an artificial color scale, especially when they are upside down and left/right reversed. . . .

Pay particular attention to the hot spot at the base of the image and note how it can appear "hot," "cold" or "disappear" depending on the color scale used. (Murphy 1996)

Murphy and Ter Pogossian both describe the danger in attempting to actually read a PET image out of context. Their discussions highlight the tension between what semiologist Jacques Bertin has referred to as *elementary* (and intermediate) readings of graphic images—in which the image is analyzed internally for relations between elements or groups of elements—and the *overall* reading, in which the image is apprehended as a whole, a gestalt impression, or in gross comparison to another image. An elementary reading of a PET image, for example, would involve attempting to determine the flow rate for a particular anatomical area, by attempting to read the value for a particular pixel as the flow rate for the voxel. An intermediate reading would involve comparing one hemisphere with another, or the value of a ROI in one image with the same ROI in another. These distinctions in reading practices concern how "technologies of representation" are deployed by scientists and others to build persuasive accounts about the structure of natural and social worlds. This is what Lynch and Edgerton called aesthetics, "the very fabric of realism: the work of discriminating difference, . . . and establishing evident relations" (Lynch and Edgerton 1988).[39] PET is a particularly good case to examine in this regard because the data it provides is so interdisciplinary and expert, yet its images also appear quite convincing to nonexperts as well. In addition to color schemes, there are also completely different conventions for representing the data as brain images. The examples in the color plate section give an idea of the difficulty of reading images across labs.

Extreme Images

Once the data has been condensed into a series of images and analyzed, the researchers must decide which images to publish. In the following discussion, a researcher comments on the process of using PET images in his own articles. The image is one part of an argument that necessarily includes a textual component.

DUMIT: When you do an article on PET for a journal . . .

TER-POGOSSIAN: I'm working on one right now!

DUMIT: And you are trying to select images for the article to demonstrate one way or another what is going on. It looks to be the case — and I can't tell because often there is not that much information presented about why these two images were chosen — it looks to be the case that the most extreme images are chosen.

TER-POGOSSIAN: Sure.

DUMIT: I'm curious about this. Is this a kind of heuristic idea, that these images display the difference that is being talked about? Are they representative?

TER-POGOSSIAN: Well, it varies. It depends on how you show the images. For example, if indeed you want to emphasize a difference, you show the extreme cases. However, in any responsible article, it behooves you to emphasize also the overlapping areas — and these are in any kind of study that involves, say, the comparison of something or another — it behooves one to use a statistical analysis. In most instances we have a statistician on the staff and we [ask] him, "How do we present the data?" And he in general has his own approach; I'm not a very good statistician myself. And he gives you that data.

But to get back to what you are saying, very often indeed, in most instances you are going to select images that emphasize your case, sure. But also, you might, if you so wish, show images that on the contrary show a false positive. It depends on what you want to do. But yes, you select the images that prove your case. However, the case is also proven, supposedly, in your text.

Ter Pogossian emphasizes how extreme images — images that look the most different from each other — may be used to imply that there are significant differences that are demonstrated in the text. Alternately, an image may be used to imply that in spite of a significant finding, there remains a strong possibility of mistaking a normal case for an abnormal one. In spite of this, as he indicates, extreme images are often used.

For example, in looking at PET images in a scientific article, I was struck by the way extreme images were presented as iconic proof of significance in an experiment. In this experiment, an attempt to measure the effects of aging on the brain, forty normal volunteers, ages 18 to 78 years, were scanned with PET (figure 3.10a). A series of graphs accompanied the article produced as a result of this experiment. The caption reads: "The degree of metabolic hyperfrontality varies considerably among normal subjects, but on average declines gradually with age" (Kuhl et al. 1982). The graphs show that although the averages for

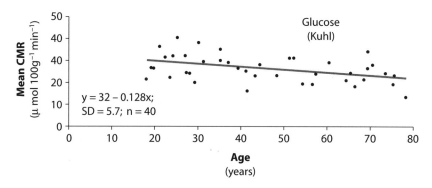

FIGURE 3.10 (a). Aging Graph. "Graph showing decline in cerebral glucose utilization (CMRglu) with age is the same in mean overall cortex, caudate-thalamus, and white matter. Each data point represents the average measurements from 5 normal subjects. Error bars represent 1 standard deviation." (From Kuhl et al. 1982, with permission)

groups of five subjects does decline, the typical variation for any age category actually overlaps the averages of every other category. In other words, given another PET scan of an unknown subject near any of the averages, there would be no basis for deciding which age category that person belongs in.

In spite of this constraint, exactly two PET images are presented in the text that look quite different from each other; one is of a 27-year-old and the other is of a 75-year-old (figure 3.10b). They were chosen not because they represented the youngest and the oldest in the set, nor because they were the average, but because they were the most extreme cases, the "extremes of [the] ratio" (Kuhl et al. 1982). In this case, the two most visibly different images of a set are presented as if representative of two different types of brains.[40] I asked one of the researchers about this:

> DUMIT: In the article, there are only two images shown, and it says underneath that these images were chosen because they were the most extremely different. Is that a standard practice, to choose the most extreme images rather than, say, the average for each?
>
> PHELPS: Yes. What is maybe not so common a practice is to point out that you did that. . . .
>
> DUMIT: Right.
>
> PHELPS: Well, yes. If you are honestly and forthrightly trying to show something in the article, you try [to] take the data and the images and process them to point that what you know to be true you can

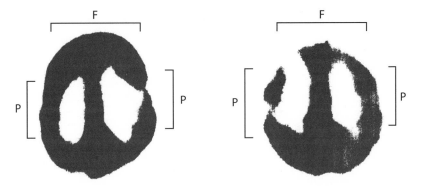

FIGURE 3.10 (b). Extreme images of aging. "The hyperfrontality index was the ratio of cerebral metabolic rate for glucose in the surperior frontal cortex (F) to the average rate in the superior parietal cortex (P). Extremes of this ratio were at 1.22 in a 27-year-old subject (left) and 0.82 in a 75-year-old subject (right)." (From Kuhl et al. 1982, with permission)

see. So we take the extreme cases for the readers to be able to see them. You have the tabulated data to look at all cases. It is fine.

Embedded in his explanation is a twofold critique: On the one hand, having carried out the experiment, the expert knows that there is a significant finding in the data. He or she can see it in the numbers, yet others, nonexperts, cannot. The expert, however, can produce a picture, using some of the data, that illustrates what the data as a whole show — an ideal to represent a statistical trend. On the other hand, this researcher is careful to note a potential abuse lurking in this practice, that the part may be taken for the whole. In this case, without the careful caption and without the accompanying data graphs, it would be easy to conclude that younger brains are *simply* quite distinguishable from older ones. It should be noted that though choosing to print extreme images appears to be standard practice, in practice such a choice is almost never stated. Researcher, Richard Haier concurred:

> We always publish group statistical data — usually analysis of variance, sometimes multiple t-tests. That is always reported in detail in the paper. Our conclusions are based on the statistics. Most of the time, although not all of the time, we include a color picture, because journals like color pictures, everybody likes color pictures — and that is what they remember. When we do that, we select images that illustrate the group statistical finding. It is not the other way around. So the picture that was in *Newsweek*, I just took the person with the highest score and the person with the lowest score [see Plate 7]. And

it looked so compelling, but that's what the effect was, that is why it was so compelling. I took the best exemplar, I took the best pair, to exemplify that. That is true. But I don't see anything wrong with that.

The images presented in these popular and scientific articles are then *not* to be carefully interpreted pixel by pixel. The displayed images should *not* be measured; they are not meant to be. Rather, they are consciously selected to enhance the textual argument. They are crafted to undergird, teach, and illustrate the process of discursive and statistical persuasion. One researcher has commented that

> Functional information is communicated very approximately by images and requires quantification to be meaningful. Thus the imaging capabilities of PET, which derive from the mode of data collection, can at best serve as an aide memoir, or illustration, of much more detailed data pertaining to a variety of cerebral functions. (Frackowiak 1986, p. 25)

Despite such qualifications, however, it is precisely these simplified "illustrations" that are valorized when these images travel from the laboratory into articles and into popular culture. In textbooks, as well, extreme images can have cultural effects. Used as illustrations of types of brains, these images become "classic" expressions of pathology, or "textbook images." In the "Chairman's Corner," an editorial spot in the journal *Investigative Radiology*, Melvyn Schreiber comments on social conditioning with which medical students learn to identify "beautiful" pictures:

> We don't mean that it's pretty but rather that it is exquisitely representative of the classic expression of the disease. When our mental conception of the textbook picture of an abnormality is reproduced perfectly in life, we describe the image as beautiful, largely out of appreciation for its verisimilitude and partly out of recognition of the ease with which the diagnosis can be made when all of the necessary elements are present and recognizable, as they so rarely are. (Schreiber 1991, p. 771)

The verisimilitude that Schreiber refers to is the fidelity of the observed image to the textbook image. The practice of producing extreme images is also encouraged by regulatory agencies and pharmaceutical companies. One researcher who had worked at a large pharmaceutical company, for instance, told of how he had to search "until the ends of the earth" to find two images, one normal and one pathological, which could clearly show the difference to the FDA. Another researcher commented on these and other popular uses of difference images:

Well, we put a lot of emphasis in trying to get pharmaceutical contracts when we started. And I think it was our experience in general that they weren't terribly interested. They were only interested at certain stages of development. If they thought it would help them get through the FDA, then they would be interested, but we found that most of our pharmaceutical contracts really came through the PR departments, the advertising departments, not through the science departments. And they were after pretty pictures to put in the ads, which apparently worked, and worked well.

I cite these examples in order to demonstrate the persuasiveness of this visual practice of exemplary images whose purpose is easy recognizability (in spite of the rarity of such recognition in practice), yet whose function is often one of proof of difference.

The risk that these picture pose, I am arguing, lies in their multivocal readings. They are both veridictory graphs and emphatic illustrations. This risk appears in stark outline in courtrooms, as discussed in chapter 4 ("Ways of Seeing Brains as Expert Images"), where the exemplary images of the most normal and most abnormal can be transformed into types, into typical representatives of normal and abnormal, to "make clear the difference." Such a process, although scientifically and legally sanctioned, risks making it appear as if one could go from single scan to diagnosis, from picture to text.

PET as a Difference Engine

In the presentation of the search for biological correlates of schizophrenic diagnoses, this collapse of scan to diagnosis seems to predominate when the correlates are located in the brain. Even though research since the 1970s has shown many relationships between this diagnosis and symptom relief through pharmacological treatment, visual presentation of "schizophrenia" seems to promise much more (Buchsbaum et al. 1985). In figure 3.11, taken from a book chapter on functional imaging, again the brain images shown are the most extreme, leaving a visual sense of clear differentiation of normal people and those with schizophrenia, even though there are many schizophrenic people whose brains look like those of normal people, and normal people whose brains look like those of schizophrenic people.[41] Significant in terms of the virtual community of images is the way in which, though the brain scans of the diagnosed normal volunteers are labeled *normal controls*, the brain scans of the diagnosed schizophrenics are labeled *schizophrenia*.[42] The image is thus labeled as showing the "disease" itself,

100

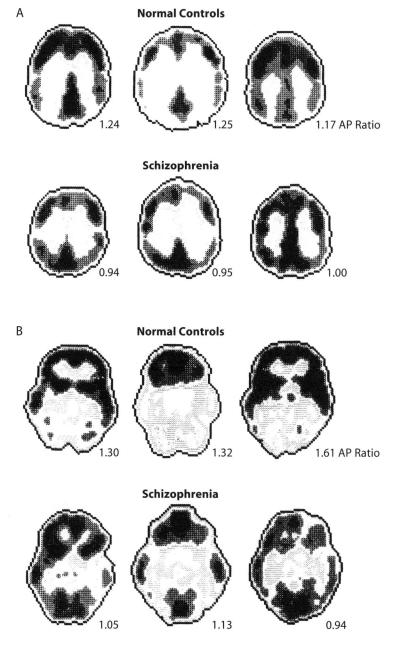

FIGURE 3.11. Schizophrenia extremes. PET supraventricular slices (a), and PET intraventricular slices (b), for three normal subjects and three patients with schizophrenia. (From Buchsbaum et al. 1985; reproduced with permission)

rather than a correlate symptom of someone found to have schizophrenia. Hence, the symptom has been collapsed into the referent.

The important danger of this collapse is that the symptom, the brain scan, should have a very complex referent. The following is a list of possible confounders, or variables that are often not taken into account but *might* affect the results of the study significantly. This list was generated from a short list of articles on PET and mental illness[43]:

Time of day, failure to control for gender and age differences, degree of handedness, position of females in their menstrual period, variations in diagnostic criteria [*Diagnostic and Statistical Manual of Mental Disorders*, third edition (*DSM*, III), vs. Research Diagnostic Criteria of Spitzer et al. (1975)], exclusion principles for comorbid conditions, behavioral phenomenology, small subject populations, psychotropic drug effects, differing experimental designs, state versus trait distinctions, metabolic and modeling assumptions, resolution versus size of anatomical areas of interest, data collection, image analysis, metabolic consequences of experimental conditions (resting, stimulations), definitions of resting, accuracy precision and reproducibility of reconstructed data, head positioning, assumptions of direct coupling of blood flow and energy metabolism, assumption that these latter two measure the same processes, assumption that subjects with illness exhibit a pattern of regular energy metabolism that can distinguish them from "normal subjects," acute/chronic differences in schizophrenia, positive and negative symptoms, duration of illness, premorbid adjustments, attentional and cognitive deficits, cycling patterns of psychosis/relative normality may not be captured or reproducible with 30-minute glimpses of metabolism, effects of diet and stress . . .

The status of these confounders in PET experiments for PET researchers is rhetorically the contrary of that used by critics of schizophrenia research. Critics such as Estroff (1993), Boyle (1990), Szasz (1987), and Rose et al. (1984) use the existence of confounders to argue against the coherence of biological explanations of schizophrenia.[44] By showing that statistically significant results *could* have originated from selection or sociological factors instead of genes, for instance, these critics contend either that there is no proof yet of biological schizophrenia or that there is in fact no such coherent category of "schizophrenia."

Were these critics to turn their analytical skills to PET studies, they would find their work already done for them. Review articles on schizophrenia list not only different findings but also contradictory ones![45] In some studies, for example, "hypofrontality" is found, meaning that the front part of the brain is less active than the rest. In other studies, "hyperfrontality" is found, meaning that the frontal lobes are more active. And in yet other studies, no difference in the frontal lobes was found. "No consistent, reproducible finding has been reported in over fifty studies," the critics might argue; "clearly here is as much proof as possible of the incoherence of the category, or of its social and not biological cause."[46]

Such reasoning, however, is not likely for neuroscientific researchers. However much they disagree about what is important about schizophrenia and what is important about the brain, they share the *Idea* that the brain must *be* in some fundamental way the person.[47] The questions, of course, are: How much of the person is discoverable from studying the brain alone? In what ways does the person exceed his or her brain?

Sublime Brains, Sublime Scans

> Once we are able to insert a molecule inside the brain, and to watch what happens to this molecule, basically the sky's the limit. I believe that PET's the reason why conventional medicine is going to transform into molecular medicine.
> — Researcher

I use the word *Idea* above in the Kantian sense of a schema through which humans understand the world. I am interested in how Kant connected conceptual processes with affective ones. In the mystery of divergent brain findings about schizophrenia, then, I suggest that neuroscience researchers find a *sublime* object, which Kant would describe as producing negative pleasure: "In presenting the sublime in nature, the mind feels agitated . . . this agitation can be compared with a vibration, i.e., with a rapid alternation of repulsion from and attraction to, one and the same object" (Kant 1987, p. 257). Negative pleasure imposes a feeling of admiration and respect. If this is the case, we can imagine the frustration and disgust with which PET researchers face the current inability to reproduce results with schizophrenic subjects and at the same time the exciting challenge presented by this inability to rationally comprehend how schizophrenia is working in the brain.

The *quality* of the feeling of the sublime consists in its being a feeling, accompanying an object, of displeasure about our aesthetic power of judging, yet of a displeasure that we present at the same time as purposive. What makes this possible is that the subject's own inability uncovers in him the consciousness of an unlimited ability

103

which is also his, and that the mind can judge this ability aesthetically only by that inability. (Kant 1987, p. 258)

For the PET researcher, the scan shows what the researcher cannot yet imagine. The scan holds a key to the mystery of schizophrenia, but the researcher cannot yet grasp it. Facing this challenge, then, taking on the job of turning contradictory results into complex understanding, might be said to be the negative pleasure of the neuroscientists. This might help in understanding their response to their so far inadequate results. The following, for example, is the conclusion of an article listing many of the confounders cited above:

> With all of the caveats and criticism noted above, we still believe that the application of PET technology to psychiatry has its brightest moments ahead. This is because we are dealing with a biochemical tool which is limited mainly by the ingenuity of the practitioners and their skill at isolating a particular brain function in an experimental paradigm. (Smith and Brodie 1986, p. 46)

The confounders, in other words, become reasons for the contradictory results. The challenge lies in lining them up so as to comprehend the whole picture, the whole scan. In some cases, the researchers substitute the truth of the image for the truth of the categories they started with. Critiquing the specificity of DSM-III-R (DSM-III, revised) and the *Diagnostic and Statistical Manuals* in general, for instance, Faulstich and Sullivan (1991) suggested that

> Significant patient heterogeneity can exist within diagnostic categories. . . . In the future, diagnostic subtypes based on PET data should be considered. Patients with a particular characteristically abnormal PET profile could be studied for patterns in genetic, biochemical, and symptomatic presentations. Groups selected in this way may be more homogeneous and may be more likely to have the same biological etiology than patient groups obtained through standard diagnostic criteria.

These PET-selected groups will be more homogeneous in their brain metabolisms. If this leads to better treatment response prediction, then this might be a good approach. In any case, the brain has become for them a receding horizon of answers.[48] Or, as another researcher put it, connecting progress in techniques to progress in solving the brain,

> [u]sing the in vivo tools of modern neuroscience, we can create comparison maps of brain terrain for diseases such as schizophrenia, bipolar disorder, major depression, Alzheimer's disease, panic disorder, autism, eating disorders, or attention deficit hyperactivity disorder

(ADHD). As has been described [in this book] this process is already well underway. During the next several decades, we can expect to identify the abnormalities in brain geography and topography that define the various types of mental illnesses. Once this is accomplished we will know where the enemy is. The techniques of molecular biology will give us the capacity to do precision bombing, while our maps of brain terrain will give us the targets at which to aim." (Andreasen 2001, p. 320)

Where critics see proof of no proof, neuroscientists see the need for more research.

In summary, PET images that appear must meet a contradictory set of demands that are satisfied by images and their justifications:

- Images are shown because they can be shown, because they are maps as much as statistics, because they symbolize and index location.
- Images are shown to illustrate the statistics, not as proof of types, but as examples of the trend and as harbingers of the kind of results that can be achieved.
- Images are icons of the ability to get information out of the brain. In the face of so many unanswered and unanswerable questions at this time, scientists need to show the ability to get results. Some thing must to be shown, as indicating current success and as indicating progress.
- Images are shown to sell the process — to get grants, to demonstrate ability before the public, to show that better results are "on the way," given more research.

In the next chapter, we will begin to look at how images circulate beyond the lab and beyond the scientific journal article. Given images of difference, what do these images mean to nonproducers, to laypeople? What kind of authority and objectivity do they have, and where? How are they read?

Dumit: Some of the places where violence [as biologically caused]
comes up are in courtrooms where PET scans have just started to
make their appearance.

Wagner: Well, there are certain general patterns that are true historically. First of all, some physicists have said, and I think quite
frankly, that every time a physical measurement is made and a
physical fact is learned, physicians try to apply it to diseases, they
try [to] relate it somehow or other to diseases, either models or
things. And I think that every time you make a correlation between
behavior and mental function, you are going to find people that are
using it in the context of free will or lack of free will. And I think it
is probably abused more than it is being used; it is probably being
misused. Some people believe that you really don't have much free
will, and will defend people on that basis. And therefore they
search for anything that can be used to support that position. They
may be right. I think it is more from a philosophical basis that they
are arguing, using that as a basis, as a tool, rather than that is a
great discovery. I mean, I'm [more] willing to believe that the person can't really control their behavior as a result of their past experience or genes than I am to say because their corpus collosum is
20 percent thicker than anybody else's, that that is the reason why
they are doing all of these things. So it's a gimmick.

Dumit: So have you testified in court?

WAGNER: I've been asked to do it. Usually we get a call here — some lawyer calls up and wants us to do a study on some person, a head-trauma patient or something like that, and I refer him to somebody else.

DUMIT: One of the fascinating cases that I found, one of the early trials using X-rays in the early 1900s, the argument before a state supreme court was: Should X-rays be shown to the jury? The claim by radiologists was that X-rays were their professional domain, one had to be trained to be able to read a radiological image. Why should the jury see the image? Because then they will eventually decide on what they think the image looks like. That seems to be one of the questions with PET scans: If they are an expert image, if they are an image that takes a lot of expertise to look at, how much does the image show, looking at it from the jury standpoint and the lay public standpoint?

WAGNER: Well, you raise an interesting question. I was raising the question of should you use the data or should you not use the data, and you are asking who should interpret the data, and that is a very interesting thought. Again it is not a question of black or white. I think there are some things that are so obvious that you don't need more expertise than the average layperson can have to interpret it. A guy who has a broken leg is an example.

DUMIT: Even though [in the early 1900s] it [was] precisely the broken leg that [was] at issue [in one of the first trials where X-rays were used]?

WAGNER: Okay. So I think that there are some technical data that it doesn't take more than the average person's intelligence to see whether it shows what is claimed to be shown. So I think you definitely should show it to the jury. It is like anything else — you don't understand English, you don't understand a person's confession. It's like saying only English majors should be able to hear confessions. I said something, did the person really confess or not confess — it depends on the meaning of their words. Since English teachers are experts on the meaning of words, you have to be a semanticist to tell the jury what the person says. All that I think is that you should not be limited in what you should show to the jury. . . . It should be up to them, whether they believe the expert or not, whether they can see it for themselves or whether they have to take the expert's word for it. And the judge helps them do it.

DUMIT: The counterargument that was proposed was that instead of English majors, it was that the juries were non-English speakers who were taught English in the court so that they could understand the confession. How much nuclear medicine do you have to be taught to understand the image?

WAGNER: It depends on the study and the result for how complicated it is for the jury to be instructed properly by the experts. And whether they are taking it on faith or whether they can really see it. "You see that this is bigger than that," and they have criteria for size and length and they take it on faith that this is not supposed to be bigger than that. But anyway, I think that you have to be very conscious that you don't misuse that information. That is what is happening right now with DNA in this morning's paper, that DNA is probably going to be getting a lot of people out of jail that should be out of jail. But probably, because of errors and variance, there are going to be some people that, by luck, are going to be able to get out of jail because of the five percent of the cases that fall outside of the two standard deviations. So it is like anything else — it can be abused or not used — and I think I would be very cautious that there [are] sufficient data. I think it is clearly a mind-set of trying to find anything that it really is an argument of free will or no free will, responsible or not responsible.

DUMIT: Yes, one philosopher phrased it that the law's assumption is that everyone has free will and science's assumption is that there is a cause for everything. Plus they added the fact that after you have competing experts in the courtroom, the court will defer towards independent or third-person objective "measurement" to help the court decide.

WAGNER: That is a very interesting way to put it.

Chapter 4
Ways of Seeing Brains as Expert Images

> Struggles over what will count as rational accounts of the
> world are struggles over how to see.
> (Haraway 1991, p. 194)

The Use of Scans in the Trial of John Hinckley

In 1981, in an apparent attempt to impress actress Jodie Foster, John
Hinckley shot President Reagan and five other people. In 1982, he was
brought to trial, and his attorneys mounted an insanity defense. As part
of this defense they petitioned to include CT scans, to show that Hinckley had an abnormal brain. CT scans are computer-generated digital
visualizations of a slice through the brain. In this case, the attorneys
wished to show that the CT scans revealed Hinckley's brain as "shrunken"
and "having enlarged sulci." They wished to use these images to help
prove that he was mentally diseased and therefore not responsible for
his actions (Caplan 1984). They argued that their expert witness, a psychiatrist, used the scans among other tests to diagnose Hinckley's condition and therefore the scans had to be admitted as evidence.

The judge presiding over the case treated these scans as potent objects. He initially denied their admittance as evidence. The defense attorneys persisted for 10 days, and eventually the judge relented, deeming
the scans relevant. In Hinckley's trial, the judge admitted two scans (one
taken immediately after the shooting and one a year later), but he took
many measures to prevent their potency from being realized:

After weeks of legal wrangling, and his ultimate decision to admit the scans, the judge did all he could to neutralize his decision. He refused to dim the courtroom lights during the display, and he insisted that the slides of Hinckley's scans be projected on a small screen set up across the large room from the jury. The performance had the impact of a short, poorly rehearsed, and annoying farce. In washed-out colors, the scans looked like slices of bruised and misshapen fruit. Clutching a yard-long stick, the radiologist who pointed out what was "strikingly abnormal" about the scans made the presentation even stranger. She shuffled to the screen in slippers and spoke in a trembling voice. By the end of the interlude, it was not likely that anyone in court had seen the scans as the clincher, closing the case with final proof of John Hinckley's disorder. (Caplan 1984, p. 85)

The judge's actions, the equivalent of "you may peek, but do not look," demonstrate a strong belief in visual and scientific persuasiveness. He clearly decided that though he could not deny their admission, he also could not rely on tempering instructions to the jury alone. Instead he took direct action on the appearance of the images, on how they should be shown, to offset what he felt were potentially prejudicial effects.

As lay readers, the powerful promise of images of the brain is that they purport to tell us about the mind. To the extent that such images are clear and reliable, we are tempted to take them for a fact and to let them help us decide about the person whose brain (and mind) is imaged. The use of brain imaging scans done with CT, MRI, PET, and SPECT in courts is increasing (Ader 1996), though as Rose (2000) observed,

> Present evidence thus suggests that biological and genetic defenses have largely failed to displace operative conceptions of responsibility within the practice of the criminal law in any jurisdiction. (p. 12)

This trend, especially with regard to claims that the images can aid jurors in deciding issues of insanity, competency, and neurotrauma, is opposed by most neurologists and other experts (Kulynych 1997; Mayberg 1992; Rojas-Burke 1993). Ter-Pogossian commented:

> I'm not a judge. But showing those pictures — I mean PET images — now to a jury, it doesn't make any sense whatsoever. I mean if whoever shows these pictures was given a stack of twenty pictures of perfectly normal subjects and twenty pictures of schizophrenics, and then you shuffle the pictures, [that person] wouldn't be able to stack

them, to unscramble them. Nobody can. There are some areas, hypo-frontality, which seem to be associated sometimes with schizophrenia, but it is a minefield.

Neuroimaging experts insist that scans cannot diagnose. Jennifer Kulynych, in the first legal review of neuroimaging in courts, argued that these images should be used only very conservatively alongside psychiatric testimony. She found that there is often little empirical evidence in terms of prior published results for the kinds of inferences that psychiatrists would like to attribute to neuroimages. Nonetheless, she noted, psychiatric testimony is usually granted admission, and therefore some method must be found "to manage the testimony, short of disallowing it altogether, so as to minimize the likelihood of undue prejudice" (Kulynych 1997, p. 1268). Her suggestion was that the court should adopt a "social framework" approach in which the judge assesses available empirical evidence and explicitly instructs the jury as to what the evidence shows so as to counteract the prejudicial effects of the testimony and demonstrative evidence.

Nancy Andreasen (2001) appeared to stake out a similar caution in *Brave New Brain: Conquering Mental Illness in the Era of the Genome*:

> Do [brain imaging technologies] help improve people's lives by making more accurate diagnoses or by guiding treatment?
>
> At the moment the value for either of those purposes is relatively limited. MR and functional imaging scans cannot be used to make a diagnosis, and we have no definitive laboratory markers or genetic tests, even for Alzheimer's disease. Most of these technological advances are still research tools, useful for probing into the brain or the molecular mechanisms of illnesses. All the data marshaled to date from imaging and electrophysiology are group comparisons. Groups of people with particular diagnosis are compared to healthy volunteers, and group differences are found. Such studies are very informative in telling us something about the brain mechanisms of an illness—that they may affect the frontal cortex, that they may involve distributed circuits, that they may suggest a neurodevelopmental abnormality. But these studies cannot make any specific predictions about an individual. They can only make predictions about the group. Thus, when neuroscientists or psychiatrists speak about the hypofrontality or ventricular enlargement in schizophrenia, they are not implying that every person with schizophrenia will have decreased frontal metabolic activity or big ventricles. Thus these findings are not useful at the moment either as screening or diagnostic tests. (pp. 158–159)

111

Andreason then went on to say that some clinicians think that it helps.

What Judge Parker in the Hinckley trial intuited and Kulynych acknowledged, but did not focus on, is the difficult problem of the undue persuasiveness of visual images, especially that category I want to call "expert images." Expert images are objects produced with mechanical assistance that *require* help in interpreting even though they may appear to be legible to a layperson. The paradox of expert images in a trial is that if they are legible, then they should not need interpretation, but if they need interpretation, then they probably should not be shown to juries.

In the next chapter, we will look at the circulation of brain images as expert images in popular culture. However, the *effectiveness* of these images, their effects and how they are read by magazine readers, movie viewers, and Web site visitors, is very difficult to assess. In this chapter, we use the court as a privileged site of explicit lay reasoning. We acknowledge with Rose that "biological arguments seem to enter the courtroom not because legal personhood has become biological, but because defense lawyers, especially in the US, utilize anything they can to defend their clients" (Rose 2000, p. 13). Judges, lawyers, and juries are laypeople with respect to brain images. They have little or no familiarity with the complex processes discussed in the previous chapter or with functional anatomy.

This chapter focuses on court decisions because this is the one area where the *power* of brain images to persuade people of form and where fact *has* to be delineated. Although there are many specific differences within the U.S. judicial system, between federal and state courts, and different kinds of trials, we can also understand the courts as a place where the persuasive, authoritative, and reifying powers of images are explicitly defined and debated in rigorous ways. By providing a survey of historical instances in which images were granted admission or censored in one way or another, a theory of the *power to make images objective* can be developed.

As we will see, even x-ray images cannot be *simply* apprehended—even by radiologists. One must learn to see them as representing the unseen, and then one can learn to interpret them for their content. In a courtroom, however, where a nonexpert audience is told what the image shows, that audience is going to be told that it illustrates a state of affairs. Here the image's apparent picture-like status and manufactured objectivity threatens to overwhelm its interpreted nature. In the courtroom, as in popular culture, the *familiarity* of the image, its *apparent* legibility, must be accounted for. These expert images are presented as doubly significant: both scientific data and socially full of meaning.

Facing images produced under scientific authority, a judge must first take into account how he or she is persuaded him- or herself of their meaning, and then how a jury might be persuaded. The judge must often make an argument as to why or why not a particular image may be shown to a jury, how it may be presented and by whom, and what referents may be attributed to it. At stake is the particular form of objectivity that an image comes to have: Is it part of an expert's *opinion*, does it indicate a *probable* relation to a fact, or is it a direct *picture of the truth*?

Courts thus directly debate the mechanisms by which images persuade and, in so doing, provide us with a set of frames for describing the visual power of brain images, and how reliant the images are on their context and form of presentation. The specific use of expert images I am concerned with in this chapter are brain images when they are used in psychiatric testimony. To understand how and why they play such an important role today, however, it is important first to look at the emergence of the category of expert images in the court in the early twentieth century with photographs and x-ray images, then to see how this notion of expert image comes to be applied to CT images and PET scanning.

Brain imaging's power comes to be a combination of scientific and medical authority, machinic and now digital objectivity, as well as cultural norms and social desirability. In many cases, ironically, this persuasiveness comes to exceed the authority and even ability of the image's authors: The very experts who made them can no longer delimit what they mean. This situation is produced, in fact, by the extreme imaging selection practices outlined in chapter 3.

X-Rays in the Courtroom

In 1896, X-rays defined the expert image of an invisible world. What is a jury supposed to do with such an expert image, however? Supposedly, as laypersons, jury members have never seen it before, nor anything like it. Yet in the courtroom, they are guided by exceedingly simple instructions, such as: Note how this part looks bigger, looks like a fracture, is shrunken, or has more holes. What I want to do is query the history of attempts to deal with this strange new creature, a visualization of an invisible world that half familiar and half alien.

Immediately popular, X-rays attracted an intense interest both inside and outside the courtroom (Golan 1999). In the first case in the United States, the question arose as to whether a radiograph or X-ray purporting to show a hip fracture could be admitted. The defendant's attorney argued against it, saying that, "the radiograph was a photograph of an object unseen by the human eye. There was no evidence that the photograph actually portrayed and represented the object pictured" (Halperin 1988, p. 640). In accepting the visual photographic metaphor, however, the attorney seemed to have sealed his fate. Judge Lefevre responded to this argument by deferring both ontologically and epistemologically to the question of history:

> We [the court] have nothing to do or say as to what [the radiographs] purport to represent; that will, without doubt, be explained by eminent surgeons. These exhibits are only pictures or maps, to be used in explanation of a present condition, and therefore are secondary evidence and not primary. They may be shown to the jury as illustrating or making clear the testimony of experts. . . . Modern science has made it possible to look beneath the tissues of the human body, and has aided surgery in telling of the hidden mysteries. We believe it to be our duty in this case to be the first, if you please, to so consider it, in admitting in evidence a process known and acknowledged as a determinant science. The exhibits will be admitted as evidence. (*Smith* v. *Grant* 1896; see Halperin 1988, p. 640)

In essence, the judge decides to defer the meaning of the x-ray images to experts while nonetheless allowing these images to be shown to juries in the manner of pictures or maps. In this sophisticated deferral, x-ray imaging is fused to the two most powerful imaging discourses: photography and cartography.

Jennifer Mnookin (1998) has traced how this precise category of "demonstrative evidence" arose in the context of photographs in the courtroom. *Demonstrative* implies that the evidence is secondary and not primary and therefore can be used only to illustrate the testimony of experts. Mnookin showed how photography, in fact, challenged courts to come up with a conceptual place that acknowledged the persuasive power of the photos but kept them off the central stage of deciding the facts of the matter. Photos were stuffed into an older analogy of maps and diagrams and granted the ability to illustrate. In fact, however, they often corroborated and persuaded. Photography's mechanical, objective nature exceeded the analogy of illustrative diagrams, and this overflow had no accountability with the court, except for the acknowledgment of such unduly prejudicial photos as these of murder victims and pornography (Hensler 1997; Selbak 1994).

Of course, X-rays do more than photographically represent what a human being might have seen. X-ray images purport to represent what no human could see. More than that, they produce a visible image *as if* it were of a potentially visible scene, even though the scene involves seeing everything on top of one another (an x-ray image is the sum of the densities of all of the materials that the rays pass through). X-ray images were then, and still are today, difficult to interpret precisely because they are *not* like photographs.

However, for the court in the late nineteenth century, faced with a nascent but popular x-ray community in which photographers were early adopters and photography was the dominant cultural metaphor, X-rays seemed tailor-made to fit into the analogy of photos and maps as demonstrative evidence (Golan 1998). According to Judge Lefevre, as objects produced by a "modern . . . determinate science," X-rays reveal mysteries to experts who alone can explain their meaning. At the same time, as secondary demonstrative evidence, like photos and maps, they are allowed to be shown to juries in the minor, neutral role of merely illustrating or making clear the expert's words. They are thus allowed in as doubled. They make clear what is unclear, but they do not make it clear to everyone.

The photographic analogy was overwhelming. A nonvisual object, x-ray attenuation, was translated into a visual one. The result was a special kind of photograph that all could see but only some could read. The Supreme Court of Tennessee ruled that

> New as this process is, experiments made by scientific men . . . have demonstrated its power to reveal to the natural eye the entire structure of the human body, and its various parts can be photographed as its exterior surface has been and now is. And no sound reason was assigned at the bar why a civil court should not avail itself of this invention, when it was apparent that it would serve to throw light on the matter in controversy. (*Bruce* v. *Veall* 1897, 41:455, quoted in Halperin 1988, p. 640).

In this manner, the jurors were asked to accept the visualized landscape of the interior as a simple object: an *aid* to the commentary of an expert. Image and text, however, compete uneasily for attention and priority. Though the court intended the radiographs as secondary evidence, to be used as an aid to "illustrate or make clear the testimony of experts," semiologists have noticed a historical reversal concerning photographs: "the image no longer *illustrates* the words, it is the words which, structurally, are parasitical on the image" (Barry 1997; Barthes 1987, p. 14; Flusser 1984). It is as if the picture, authorized by "experts," no longer needs them. Indeed, the legibility of radiographs was attacked unsuccessfully in two opposing ways.

According to some attorneys, though the radiograph was *like* a photograph, no one seemed to think that it spoke for itself (in the presumed manner of photographs), nor especially that it could diagnose by itself.

115

In courts, the photograph is upheld as evidence on three grounds: first when accompanied by a living witness to the scene, it is said to illustrate what the witness attests to. Second, the photograph can be a silent witness, testifying on its own behalf as if it were the eyes of witnesses, to be interpreted in turn by the jury. Third, the photograph can be a construction produced to look like a scene but without originary presence (Guilshan 1992; Hensler 1997; Mnookin 1998; Selbak 1994).

The x-ray image could not witness in any of these manners, because in spite of its privileged access to the interior of the patient, it still provided only signs or symptoms, not the injury itself. It showed previously unavailable information about the patient, but the significance of this information was up to the expert. Some attorneys therefore asked why a jury composed of nonexperts, of laypersons, should see the radiograph at all. Appearances might be significantly misleading. Citing the wide and significant variations in the x-ray images obtained, depending on precise alignment of angles, magnifications, and screens, attorneys in another case argued that

> there is really no more reason why a jury should see the skiagram [X-ray] than that there should be exhibited to them the clinical thermometer, stethoscope, measuring tape, and chemical apparatus, etc., used in cases which become subjects of judicial investigation. (Stover 1898, cited in Halperin 1988, p. 642)

The skiagram or radiographic image is here equated not with the injury, which would be immediately relevant, but with instrument readings and streams of numbers. In other words, the radiograph is argued to be a code; and codes can be deceptive. Jury members, might decide that something that *looked like* a fracture, for instance, to their untrained eyes might be a fracture. Though codes might appear to *be* cognizable objects, these code-images can be deciphered and interpreted only by experts. They do not merely magnify or make the invisible visible; they are transforming or translating a nonvisual set of relations into a specialized visual object.

Other attorneys posed the opposite analogy, arguing that radiographs are not so deeply coded. Perhaps x-ray images are simply better eyes, rather than different ones. If the code is not so difficult to master, then perhaps jurors' judgment can be partially severed from that of the experts. In a leg-fracture case in 1896, attorneys "argued that the expert witness should only have been allowed to explain what, in general, constituted a fracture on a radiograph and leave it for the jury to determine from the exhibited film whether or not a fracture was present" (Halperin 1988, p. 641). Here they treated the radiograph like a photograph, one that the jury is able to read and understand with minimal orientation. If jury members can be taught, however, then the expert should step aside and let the jury members form their own opinions as to the meaning of the object portrayed.

These two critiques of the use of X-rays as expert images founder on the instability of the category of demonstrative evidence as *merely* illustrating and making clear the testimony of experts. On the one hand, if the image is readable with minimum orientation, like a map or a photo, then the jury should be allowed to draw its own conclusions as to the relation between the image and the testimony. On the other hand, if the image is legible only to a highly trained expert, the only function of showing it to the jury would be to play on its commonsensical, but wrong, notions as to what the image *should* look like. The courts rejected both of these arguments, insisting on the scientific guarantee of the veracity of the process of representation that produced the radiograph. This guaranteed veracity produced them as *mere* aids and illustrations to the text, and as such, it was agreed that they were not harmful but were in most cases helpful.

This discussion of X-rays makes clear some parameters of visual persuasion at stake in contests over the power of visualization. For the rest of this chapter, I will be considering contemporary imaging technologies, CT and PET scanning, whose status in court, in clinical medicine, and in many disciplines of science is still being debated.

CT Images Are Like X-Ray Images

Looking today at CT scans in the mass media, we find familiar the brain-like shapes in black and white. Henry Wagner described the arrival of the CT scan in terms of the "shock of recognition" of seeing the brain (Wagner 1986). Most contemporary understandings of the CT scan assume it to unproblematically represent the structure of the brain, even if it does not do so as well as MRI in most cases. However, as histories of the x-ray image have shown, even images that today seem obviously recognizable were themselves the subject of acculturation (Pasveer 1989; Reiser 1978; Reiser and Anbar 1984). Eco (1979) stated this problem succinctly: "Similarity does not concern the relationship between the image and its object, but that between the image and a previously culturalized content" (p. 204) This insight is not always obvious. That recognition is a social process and not inherent came as a surprise, for example, to the marketing department of EMI, the company that first developed the CT scanner:

PHELPS: An extreme case was when the CAT [computerized axial tomography] scanner came out. The entire marketing department of

117

EMI, who made the CAT scan, went through a terrible frustration, because Professor Bole, from London, had gone around showing people CAT scans of the brain that were quite remarkable, but people didn't think very much of it. And so John Bole came to America; he had to build the commercial success of the CAT scanner in America. He went around to all these radiologists showing CAT scans. He could see tumors and hemorrhages, strokes, and he was appalled by the fact that the radiologists didn't respond that well. And in fact a whole group of purported leadership of radiology in that early time projected that the world market for CAT scanners was seventeen units and that it would take ten years to get there. Seventeen units!

DUMIT: So radiologists didn't grasp the significance of CAT scans?

PHELPS: No. They had never seen the brain. Neurosurgeons had. They opened up the skull and they looked in there. They looked at the CAT scan and they said, "I know I've seen that. That is the brain. And there is a lesion in reference to all these major sulci." They could see the ventricles noninvasively. "These are all the classical surgical landmarks, and here is a lesion in relation to them. This is incredible."

Drs. Robert Ledley and John Mazziotta had to put together a very limited atlas at that time, showing cut sections of the cadavers and whole-body ACTA [automatic computerized transverse axial] scans of them. And although rudimentary, it was a great accomplishment. Anytime that you look at something different [from what] you've ever seen before, you've got to learn what it looks like. And you have to learn what the norm looks like, before you can say, "This is not normal." (Michael Phelps, August 4, 1993, conversation with the author, University of California, Los Angeles)[1]

Here then is an important cultural lesson in seeing, and in seeing what is "normal" and what is "not normal." To see something new, some people must figure out how to see it and then teach others. The cultural salience of the CT scans of the brain went further, however, because it traded also on the equation of the brain with psyche. For the first time (outside of large tumor detection), there was the possibility of seeing an abnormal brain rather than diagnosing an abnormal mind. The slippage between these two forms of recognition is tricky because the first necessarily relies on the second.

One cannot, for instance, actually see mental illness in the brain; one can see only the large variations in different brains and attempt to correlate certain kinds of brains with certain diagnoses — normal, schizophrenic, depressed, and so on. The desire, of course, is for the machine-imaged brain to replace the psychiatrically diagnosed mind, the "holy grail" of biological psychiatry.[2]

Thus, even though the brain images are produced by people, they are coproduced by scientific machines, and it is the machines, especially computers, that leave their mark. Scientists, as demonstrated by many researchers in science studies, increasingly attempt to remove their marks from the image, even though they must still provide the text (Daston and Galison 1992; Star 1989, 1992). At the crux of this relationship between the image that (objectively) speaks for itself and the expert who (subjectively) reads its lips is a desire by the court and by everyone else to reduce ambiguity, to make things clear, and clearly acceptable.

> Uneasy with the possible prejudice intrinsic to such capricious and judgmental factors, the courts have looked to science to provide more solid insights into human behavior. . . . Belief in the power of science to provide hard facts shapes decisions about the proper disposition of those responsible for criminal behavior. And, scientific evidence is increasingly valued as a means to enhance the efficiency and effectiveness of overcrowded courts. (Nelkin and Tancredi 1989, p. 134)

The risks of such an emphasis on clear and efficient demarcation of subjective expert and objective machine are that any of the components — the imaging process, the expert interpretation, or the concept of the brain and disease — are themselves ambiguous or multivocal and thus prematurely closed off by efficient measurements.

Demonstrating Objective Brains

> Be sure to spend adequate time with your [expert medical] witness to work out your approach and format for elevating the jury from a plane of zero knowledge on this technique to a plane of adequate knowledge so that they can interpret the demonstrative evidence which you have to offer. Remember, these newer techniques (such as the CAT scan) may be your *only* objective, demonstrative "proof" that add weight to the *subjective* opinion of your medical witnesses. This being true, make the most of it! Whether the jury accepts your "objective" evidence may determine the outcome of your entire case.
> (Houts 1985, p. 22)

119

Houts's text, the first instance I found of explicit instructions to attorneys for effectively using digital brain images, emphasizes the veridictory weight of scientific images. The process prescribed for the medical expert is one of positioning oneself as subjective guarantor of objective evidence, as fallible witness of an infallible device.

This is an explicit example of what Greimas and Courtes (1982) called *planar semiotics*, "the ways in which relative to a given culture, certain signs [are judged] to be 'more real' than others" (pp. 150–151). Semiotics is "the study of how physical properties of bodies are assumed as signs, as vehicles for social meanings" (de Lauretis 1987, p. 25). Using semiotics, we can study the material and cultural ways in which codes, bodies, and technologies are intrinsically bound up with each other. In U.S. popular and court culture, machine images, experts, and diagnosis are bound together in a hierarchical manner. For instance, the following series of questions was suggested by Harry Rein, M.D., J.D., for attorneys to pose to jurors when employing medical images in a courtroom:

> Is there a difference between objective and subjective, and if so, what is that difference? Is a thermogram objective? Would it help the jury understand your answers if you showed some of the thermograms? Please describe those to the jury. (Rein 1986, p. 119)

Rein called for attorneys to define for their juries different *levels* of realness and then to situate images, people, and processes in relation to them. In the case of these scientific medical visualizations, objectivity must first be presented as different from and even the opposite of subjectivity. Second, objectivity must be presented as better than subjectivity. Finally, scientific visualizations must be connected to the former and divorced from the latter.

What these passages make clear is that medical images are seen by attorneys as capable of demonstrating far more power, objectivity, and truth than the "mere illustration and making clear" of demonstrative evidence. Expert brain images come to be seen as making the facts visible and being the only objective "proof" that grounds rather than supplements the expert's truth. Semiotically, we can see that rather than there being a need for agreement on the chain of representations before logic and rationality can be secured, the rationality and logic of the digital images are being invoked to secure agreement. Ted Porter, for instance, has studied the forms of trust that quantification enables in different settings. Drawing on science studies work, including Steven Shapin and Simon Schaffer's *Leviathan and the Air-Pump* (Shapin and

Schaffer 1985), Porter described one of the relationships between a democratic state and quantification in the following manner:

> It is not by accident that the authority of numbers is linked to a particular form of government, representative democracy. Calculation is one of the most convincing ways by which a democracy can reach an effective decision in cases of potential controversy, while simultaneously avoiding coercion and minimizing the disorderly effects of vigorous public involvement. (Porter 1992, pp. 28–29)

Porter examines how, within policy studies, the ability to produce quantitative results provides a rallying point within a bureaucratic democracy. Numbers do this work because they are repeatable and because they are nonsubjective and thus disinterested.

> [T]he crucial point is that faith in the objectivity of quantitative methods is not quite the same thing as the acceptance of the validity of their conclusions. The "objectivity" of quantitative policy studies has more to do with their fairness and impartiality than with their truth. (Porter 1992, p. 29)

In this planar semiotics of democracy, truth depends at least as much on social consensus as on true correspondence. The fair, impartial objectivity of numbers is more persuasive, or "harder," than the partial subjectivity of an expert—harder, potentially, than even the expert who produced those numbers, because the expert's subjectivity is inherently linked to bias. Some "expert" brain researchers are quite excited by this possibility in the courtroom: "Another advantage of 'behavioral imaging' [based on algorithmic detection of abnormalities] is the reduced need to rely on experts who were hired by one of the parties" (Gur and Gur 1991, p. 181). Despite their optimism regarding this automatic replacement of expertise with programming, the Gurs note that no specific pattern has been established for any psychiatric disorder. Nonetheless, they state that "when such diagnostic markers are established [for schizophrenia], diagnosis of insanity could be made on the basis of more objective data than is possible today" (p. 180). They thus paradigmatically conflate schizophrenia with insanity.

The suspicion of subjectivity as tainting scientific results often extends all the way down to the researcher him- or herself, where this suspicion serves as motivation to act. One PET researcher described the process of designing software to analyze PET images:

> When you saw an area of increased activity in a PET scan, it wasn't clear whether it was noise or not. And, there was enough variability in location from person to person, that it raised the possibility of

121

fudging the data. That is, you could pick a hot spot over here that was noise, and in the next subject, here is a little bit of noise over here. And if you went through and always picked the hottest spot, in any subject, kind of in a ballpark vicinity, you could then show that any area activated. And so my motivation was always to try [to] find a way to remove the potential to bias the data. That was a substantial risk, and the more that the processing could be automated and made noninteractive, the more reliable it would be, and the more replicable it would be. Since it doesn't seem that we know anything unless somebody else can replicate it, that was steadily a big push, to automate the processing.

Here, the presence of subjectivity creates a gap between the research and reality. This gap becomes the structure of the researcher's desire, motivating him to eliminate the appearance of subjectivity through automating all the tasks he presently is involved in. This researcher illustrates the taboo nature of subjectivity in science; subjectivity is seen as polluting the process of progress. Every possibility of subjectivity *must* be eliminated to produce something reliable—that is, something real, something known. The hero in this story is automation, which stands as the opposite of interactivity.

The kind of automation that the researcher turns to is computing, or "embodied calculation" in Porter's terms. The computer can reduce bias and therefore produce consent because it is so "dumb." In the language of democracy, if "even a thing as stupid as a computer" (Porter 1992, p. 644) can produce the image, then there can be no individual advantage or subjective bias involved. The resulting image is therefore neutral and can produce democratic consensus.

Mark Mintun, PET researcher at Washington University, stated:

> Lots of people talk about PET being able to map the brain. . . . They take a single picture of the brain at rest or doing something, and they say, You see this area over here? This is what I think is going on." The science is very weak. It's nice for pictures, but the real bottom line is it's guesswork. (Froelich 1987, p. 17)

He then goes on to state how they automated the process so that "there's no question whether you see it or whether the person responded. It's just not guesswork anymore."[3]

In concluding this section, I must note that I am not trying to throw suspicion on the process of automation. Instead, I am attempting to reconstruct the consequences of this particular objective, normalizing, and democratic notion of automation. This automation is inherently antisubjective and antivariable, and ironically, it therefore becomes anti-expert. One particularly difficult anti-expert bind comes up in malpractice suits involving machines. For instance, Gagliardi (1988) commented, "I mourn the damage done to the profession by those who started describing CT scanners as being first generation or second generation. The implication of superiority, regardless of skill of the operator, is apparent" (p. 1988, 636). *Inferior* (because a machine is older or has lower resolution) translates too easily into *inferior care* and *inferior experts* in a manner analogous to automatic machines equaling supreme expertise.[4] The expert craft at the base of scientific practice and the experienced art at the base of neuromedical interpretation are covered over and even denigrated in the name of neutral clarity.[5]

Insanity by Machine

> Today CAT scans and NMR scans and drug therapies
> are used in the diagnosis and treatment of behavioral
> disorders. The concept of a sick brain replaces that of the
> sick mind. . . . I argue that behavior is controlled by the
> brain, even those behaviors with which lawyers deal, and
> we must reinterpret such legal concepts as insanity and
> free will into physical, neurological concepts. Medical
> definitions must replace legal definitions.
> (Jeffery 1994, pp. 172, 174)

The adjudication of insanity by the courts is a long-standing and vexing problem. At issue are social as well as individual causes of human action, and the relation of the causes to the legal question of guilt or innocence. *Evil or Ill?*, Lawrie Reznek's masterful review of the processes through which judges and juries determine guilt and innocence when the quality of the defendant's mind is questioned, reveals a surprising conclusion. Despite the long debates, treatises, hearings, and laws on the matter of how to define and prescribe the determination of insanity, judges and juries often decide not on rules but on everyday notions: did the person know what he or she was doing? Further, juries' decisions regarding insanity are mediated by their assessment of the character of the defendant. Reznek terms this "evil or ill." In practice, he claimed, if the defendant is guilty but basically good, then he or she is more likely to be found "ill" (insane). If however, he or she is guilty and evil, then juries will tend to find them not ill but just plain evil and guilty (Reznek 1997).

Underdiscussed by Reznek is the role that might be played by biological determinations of mental disorders, especially those biomedical

123

techniques that appear unbiased and unmediated by the beliefs of a psychiatrist. Legally and socially, there is no necessary connection between an abnormal brain and an insane person (Morse 1988; Perlin 1990). However, popular portrayals of the brain continuously reiterate the chain of associations that an abnormal brain implies mental illness, which implies insanity (Gilman 1988; Dumit 1997). Lelling (1993), for example, has shown how the legal model of insanity is dependent on both the medical-biological model of mental illness and also popular models. Drawing on the work of Reisner and Slobogin, Lelling noted how the medical model presumes that "mental states result primarily from organic or chemical conditions within the human body" (Lelling 1993, n. 80; Reisner et al. 1999). The medical presumptions, which conclude (1) that the cause of behavior lies within the person, (2) that the cause is in principle verifiable, and (3) that the medical model is generally accepted, all accord well with the desires of the court. Lelling further noted that biological notions of insanity are themselves dependent on folk psychology, on the idea that the brain is integral to reason and volition and that the brain is both conditioning and irresistible (Lelling 1993).

In court, the claim by a psychiatrist that a person's schizophrenia is biologically based is still a claim or opinion that can be countered by another psychiatrist. Should evidence be proffered, however, *showing* a brain "defect" or a "visible abnormality," there arises the additional concern that such evidence might provide a "misleading aura of certainty" (*Huntington* v. *Crowley* 1966). Here judges are distinguishing between different kinds of persuasion and their relative force. Thus, even as "experts with impressive credentials" (*People* v. *Kelly* 1976) are debated regarding their effect on juries, *machines* and graphic evidence come in for even greater caution:

> When a witness gives his personal opinion on the stand—even if he qualifies as an expert—the jurors may temper their acceptance of his testimony with a healthy skepticism born of their knowledge that all human beings are fallible. But the opposite may be true when the evidence is produced by machine: like many laypersons, jurors tend to ascribe an inordinately high degree of certainty to proof derived from an apparently "scientific" mechanism, instrument, or procedure. Yet the aura of infallibility that often surrounds such evidence may well conceal the fact that it remains experimental and tentative. (*People* v. *MacDonald* 1984)

To put it explicitly, experts do not brainwash jurors the way that machines do. "Expert testimony does *not* seek to take over the jurors' task of judging credibility nor does it tell the jury that any particular witness is or is not truthful or accurate" (*People* v. *Gray* 1986). The point of these court decisions is that in some cases, technology appears to take over not only seeing but judging as well. The evidence no longer presents itself nor is received as data to be interpreted but as veridictory statements about the organization of the world.

The relationship of machine to psyche first came to a head with the Frye decision involving whether or not a polygraph, or lie detector, could be admitted into evidence (*Frye* v. *United States* 1923). The Frye case and then *Daubert* v. *Merrell Dow Pharmaceuticals, Inc.* are famous for setting out criteria for adequate scientificity of evidence. There is an added reason to exclude polygraph evidence, however. Hensler, in his comprehensive review of the admissibility of polygraphs before and after *Daubert*, documented how countless courts have excluded polygraph evidence because the prejudicial impact of admitting the results substantially outweighs their probative worth (Hensler 1997, n. 225; see notes 193–195). Federal Rule of Evidence 403 states that "Although relevant, evidence may be excluded if its probative value is substantially outweighed by the danger of unfair prejudice."

The question of prejudice arises in the case of the polygraph when the jury's judgment-making ability is taken from them. Undue prejudice is defined in the Advisory Committee's Note to Rule 403 as "an undue tendency to suggest decision on an improper basis, commonly, though not necessarily, an emotional one" (Hensler 1997, citing Federal Rule of Evidence 403 advisory committee notes). In addition to being unreliable, even though potentially helpful, "expert polygraph evidence is distinguishable from such techniques as DNA testing . . . in that only polygraphy goes directly to the ultimate issue at trial: the defendant's guilt or innocence. If believed by the jury, the expert polygraph testimony decides the case" (Hensler 1997, pp. 1293–1294). Henseler came down hard on the admission of polygraphs into the court. Even if they should satisfy *Daubert* (which he doubted), they should then be excluded as prejudicial under Rule 403.

CT scan images of the brain that purport to be about insanity or competency of a person may also be seen to go to the ultimate issue of the trial, in this case to a person's responsibility for his or her actions. Whether the brain image might be prejudicial is also a cultural question of whether a person's brain status can be equated with his or her mental status and personhood—that is, whether the jury feels that *abnormal brain = mentally ill = not responsible*. (See Masters and McGuire 1994 for one debate on this issue.) In the case of the CT scans in Hinckley's trial, once the scans were accepted as representing brains, and once

125

brains were accepted as representing states of personhood, then it was a simple, logical step to read Hinckley's rationality from the scans.

Indeed, Nancy Andreasen's 1984 account of Hinckley and schizophrenia reveals exactly this sort of logic. Her best-selling book, *The Broken Brain: The Biological Revolution in Psychiatry,* with a PET scan on the cover, compellingly argues for the visibility of mental illness through brain imaging (see Plate 13). In the following example, she concisely argues that many schizophrenic people have enlarged ventricles and so did Hinckley and that therefore, Hinckley was probably schizophrenic:

> [Figure 4.1] shows a much more common abnormality observed in schizophrenic patients. This CT scan shows two cuts from the brain of a twenty-eight-year-old man. . . . The ventricles in this man's brain are relatively enlarged for his age. . . .
>
> Both of these findings indicate that the patient's brain has shrunk and withered. . . . These types of CT-scan abnormalities, particularly ventricular enlargement, are relatively common in patients suffering from schizophrenia. John Hinckley, the young man who attempted to assassinate President Reagan, had very similar abnormalities on his CT scan.
>
> Thus many psychiatrists have begun to order CT scans frequently for those patients in whom the diagnosis of schizophrenia or dementia is likely. Many of these patients will have completely normal CT scans, but some will have the abnormalities of the type shown [here]. When these abnormalities are noted, they indicate that the patient's symptoms are probably due to a structural cause in the brain. Since ventricular enlargement is relatively common in schizophrenia, this finding may also help confirm the diagnosis of schizophrenia. John Hinckley's abnormal CT scan suggests quite strongly that he suffers from schizophrenia: Behind his abnormal behavior is an abnormal brain. (Andreasen 1984, pp. 169–171)

Andreasen's emphasis in her book was on alleviating suffering and reducing the stigma of mental illness, but her argument might as well be a court presentation of the semiotics of CT scanning and schizophrenia. We should note here the puzzling confusion over false negatives (schizophrenic patients with completely normal CT scans) and false positives (normal people with abnormal CT scans).[6] In claiming that "Hinckley's abnormal CT scan suggests quite strongly that he suffers from schizophrenia," Andreasen appeared to be concluding causality from correlation. In her argument, the correlation of person and measurement seemed to require that conclusion.

Normal brain　　　　　　　　Abnormal brain

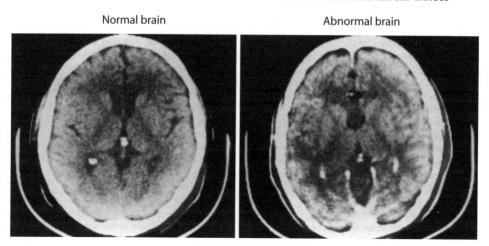

FIGURE 4.1. Scans from normal and schizophrenic patients. (From Andreasen 1984)

Judge Parker's actions in the Hinckley trial—not allowing the theory relating shrunken brains to schizophrenia because of lack of evidence and allowing the scans only at the far end of the room—demonstrate an awareness of the power of this kind of visual logic. The judge nonetheless allowed the scans to be shown to the jury as relevant. "But relevant to what?" queried Sander Gilman, testifying before Congress in the aftermath of the case:

> There was certainly no link between brain size and schizophrenia shown by psychiatry at this time. Even the defense acquiesced to this fact. Why then was it necessary to introduce this material? Because it showed that there was a potential physical cause of Hinckley's action, within his biology, not his psyche. (National Commission on the Insanity Defense 1983)

Crucially, Gilman stated that all a brain scan needs to show is a potential cause, and that thereafter jurors might make the cultural division between biology and psyche. The element of the CT scan images crucial to their potency is their visuality. They purport to show the difference between a normal and abnormal brain, between a normal person and an abnormal person, and they purport to do so scientifically and objectively. Simply put, because most of us think that the brain of an insane person *should* somehow be different from a sane person's, we hope that there is a way to detect this difference. Even more than the social and cultural stereotypes of mental illness that Gilman has so ably documented, digital brain images promise that an objective—that is, culture-

127

free — machine can distinguish *them* (the mentally abnormal) from *us* (Gilman 1988).

The Functional Brain in Courtrooms

> Brain scans can help convince a jury that something is wrong with a defendant's mind. "Most juries feel that most mental patients are really faking," explained Dr. Bernard Diamond. . . . "If you show them the X-ray, they're convinced." But prosecutors fear the colorful pictures PET scans and some EEGs produce may dazzle jurors. . . . [One attorney] said he was concerned jurors "would be staring at these pretty pictures . . . and just equate all the red colors with crazy colors."
> (DeBenedictis 1990, p. 30)

PET scans have been and continue to be controversial in courtrooms (Nelkin and Tancredi 1989; Stipp 1992). PET represents cutting-edge science; it is both experimental and a sign of progress. In addition, because its visualizations may purport to show "dramatic evidence of brain damage" (Martell 1992, p. 324), they are also potentially prejudicial. Unlike CT scanning or MRI, which show the structure of the brain and are relatively stable over time, PET's portrayals of brain functions can vary from day to day or moment to moment, depending on what a person is doing, feeling, or taking. Consequently, the ability to isolate a specific kind of impairment — mental illness, incompetency, or difficult to define neurological damage — is subject to challenge on a number of grounds. These include the specificity of the scan (Can it demonstrate a connection between this person and the impairment?), the presence of confounders (Is the person adequately normal in all other respects?), and timeliness (Is the person's brain now the same as it was during the crime?). On these grounds, most PET researchers firmly oppose the use of PET scans in a courtroom.

Because the category of expert medical image is applied to PET, the operative criterion for legal admission can shift from "Is it scientifically acceptable?" to "Can it be legitimately used by a doctor to *help* make a diagnosis?" In this section, I want to show how under this criteria, PET is often admissible if care is taken in matching the subject to the published literature and to a normal control group. In the next section, I argue that the crux of the matter is acknowledging that these are *expert* images that are simply not readable by nonexperts and that they are deeply misleading and prejudicial to show to juries.

As discussed in the previous chapter, a PET image is dynamic, manipulable, and difficult to decipher even for an expert. Yet showing it to jury members would most likely appear to help them understand how and why a doctor was able to use the PET scan in making a diagnosis. In cases in which what is at issue is a disease or disorder well discussed in the medical literature — Alzheimer's dementia or epilepsy — this is relatively unproblematic. In a number of cases, however, PET images have been admitted even when the theory connecting the images to either mental illness or insanity has not. In *People* v. *Weinstein*, a case before the Supreme Court of New York involving the use of PET scans for an insanity defense, Judge Carruthers excluded all theory but allowed that the jury should be shown the scans. He further held that "relevant evidence that does not meet the *Frye* standard may still be admissible on issue of sanity." Citing both Section 4.07(4) of the Model Penal Code and Section 60.55(1) of New York's Criminal Procedure Law, Judge Carruthers noted that psychiatrists and psychologists may use "relevant and reasonable" technical and scientific material to form diagnostic opinions that have not been accorded general acceptance within their discipline and that these materials may be shown to the jury (*People* v. *Weinstein* 1992). This decision led to a plea. Kulynych, writing against the use of neuroimages in courtrooms, accused Judge Carruthers of perhaps "being seduced by defense rhetoric and the high-tech glamour of neuroimaging" (Kulynych 1997, p. 1263). Her claim was that neuroimaging is not diagnostic and therefore should not be evidence.

The problem with this line of arguing is that it again confuses the kind of evidence that PET presents for psychiatrists. Especially in cases involving medical doctors, there is wide latitude granted to tests that are reasonably relied on to help form an opinion on the subject — in this case, diagnosis (Federal Rules of Evidence 403). Most neurologists and psychiatrists familiar with PET would agree that it can *aid* in making a differential diagnosis even though it is not in itself a reliable indicator of either morbidity or normality. In *People* v. *Weinstein*, Judge Carruthers made clear his sympathy with the auxiliary use of PET as an aid in determining a diagnosis, even if the use was purely negative, only to rule certain other possibilities.

In each of these cases, *to the extent* that PET met Daubert criteria in connection with their aid in making diagnoses, they were admitted into evidence.[7] In terms of scientificity, it will be increasingly hard to deny admission of neuroimaging data, especially when the presenters are clear about using "consistent with" language and pointing out how useful PET is in excluding other diagnoses. On the basis of my ethnographic and cultural studies approach to neuroimaging, however, I would like to strongly suggest a careful evaluation of the prejudicial nature of showing brain images to a jury. In this final section, I argue that these expert images are not simply potentially manipulated and dynamic but that their cultural familiarity merits close scrutiny of how they are received in the courtroom.

Prejudicial Images

> I was told that one judge, in pretrial, decided that he would admit PET scanning. No judge has decided that he wouldn't, but this judge decided that he wouldn't allow the jury to *see* any of the pictures. He would just allow the testimony about what was in the pictures because he felt that the pictures in themselves were prejudicial. This strikes me as absolutely true. This seems to me to be a very wise decision. Because those pictures are very compelling, and what I told the superior court justices is that if you wanted to manipulate PET, it was very hard to fake it by saying, "What can I think now to activate my left anterior thalamus?" But as an operator, I can choose the colors on the scale and I can choose the interval on the scale, and I can make a lot of areas black. And that would look very dramatic. That is about the worst thing I think one can do to make a visual presentation that was not entirely accurate.
> (Richard Haier, quoted in Dumit 1995b, p. 67)

Haier emphasizes the difference between describing a brainset and portraying it in color. The latter risks overestimating the differences involved and therefore making a slightly ambiguous statistical correlation appear to be clear and dramatic. Three issues must be unpacked in this description: (1) the status of the referent of PET images, (2) the kind of objectivity of PET scanning, and (3) the persuasiveness of such images for viewers. These issues define the kind of message that a PET scan becomes in popular culture and in the courtroom.

First, recall the customary practice of publishing extreme images outlined in the previous chapter. As an illustration of the kinds of problems that these extreme images pose, consider the following hypothetical scenario: In an experiment comparing people found to have schizophrenia with people who have no history of mental illness in their family (these are called supernormals in the literature), data is generated that shows much overlap between the two groups but enough statistical difference to warrant publication. In other words, though there is clearly no way to go from scan to diagnosis, there are certain areas of the brain that have more activity in more people with schizophrenia than in supernormals. Imaging software is used to process the brain data so as to highlight those schizophrenia-elevated areas. To make clear the difference to nonexperts, the supernormals are used to establish a baseline set of color ranges, and the average of the images is then produced. This process of averaging suppresses the many individual variations among the supernormals and produces a fairly smooth image of "normal." The average image of people with schizophrenia will have, because of the color ranges chosen, enough of a variation in a few regions to be visibly different. The schizophrenia image will thus appear to look like the normal image but with visible "defects" standing out, areas usually colored yellow, red, or black.

One approach to selecting images for display would be to take the supernormal with the most smooth scan and to publish it as NORMAL next to the scan from the person with schizophrenia whose brain regions were most different and to label that one as SCHIZOPHRENIA. The visual gestalt would be one of a clear difference between the different types of persons and the clear *visual* implications that (1) almost anyone could see schizophrenia with neuroimaging, (2) that schizophrenic people have a certain kind of brain, and (3) that schizophrenic people are clearly biologically different from normal people. Implications like these are routinely displayed in the mass media, where the accompanying text often asserts what the pictures show, not what the data originally indicated.

Now comes a semiotic problem for those researchers, such as Ter-Pogossian, who want to argue that one cannot diagnose schizophrenic images or sort them from normal ones. They want to argue that brain imaging cannot (yet) demonstrate a correspondence between a subject's scan and a diagnosis of schizophrenia. However, they are up against a claimant who argues that the image shows *clearly* visible difference, that it is an abnormal scan, defined as such for the jury by the rules of invention:

> We may define as invention a mode of production whereby the producer of the sign-function chooses a new material continuum not yet segmented for that purpose and proposes a new way of organizing (of giving form to) it in order to map within it the formal pertinent element of a content-type. . . . The sign producer must in some way posit this correlation so as to make it acceptable. (Eco 1979, p. 245)

The claimant's task is to posit that this new material continuum, the brain scan, is either visually dissimilar (or similar) to other brain scans, and that this dissimilarity is related to abnormality. On the face of it, this position seems quite acceptable: brain scan type A goes with person type A, and brain scan type B goes with person type B. We might note here that the popular media practice of publishing simply labeled brain images of extreme cases makes this interpretation all the more conventional, and hence acceptable.

The claimant who suggests that an "abnormal scan equals abnormal person" is able to define a simple, elegant organization, and one that is eminently visualizable: yellow blob versus no yellow blob. The researcher who disputes this organization is in the difficult position of arguing that the scan, *despite appearances*, is *not* simply readable (as opposed to *simply* not readable). He or she must argue that the scan is, in fact, an expert image requiring context and reflection, not reflexive speculation. The researcher must argue that even though it looks different from an "average normal" scan, there may be no (significant) difference in the person at all.[8] He or she is caught here in the sublime dilemma of brain imaging, attempting to argue that the yellow blob or any other "abnormality" might nonetheless mean that the person is "completely normal."

This kind of image publishing practice is routine in the life sciences and is in fact demanded by journals, grant agencies, and the FDA. All of these institutions, if they are to look at images, want images that are visually distinguishable, images that do not require one to be an expert to see a difference. In courtrooms, however, one of the side effects of these publishing practices is that many normal people, especially those who do not meet the criteria for supernormal, will look more abnormal than not. Normal variation will have a tendency to stand out from the averaged supernormal and look more like the published abnormal images.

Furthermore, despite the tremendous work being done with brain imaging and mental illness, there remains much difficulty in interpreting individual scans. There is as much, *if not more*, difficulty diagnosing scans than diagnosing schizophrenia using traditional psychiatric evaluations. This does not mean that neuroimaging does not aid in forming an opinion about a person regarding schizophrenia or other mental illnesses or neurological disorders. It can and does, and therefore should be admitted as evidence aiding in making a diagnosis. It does mean, however, that showing these expert images to a jury literate in only popular images of absolute differences and medical journal images of extreme and admittedly exaggerated differences is potentially prejudicial, because the jury's eyes are cultural ones, not expert ones.

If popular and extreme images accord with our cultural-commonsense notions of the differences between them (abnormals) and us (normals), as Sander Gilman has argued, how can we look at expert images of the brain and not engage our prejudices as to what we think mental illness looks like? The use of expert images in the courtroom is fraught with difficulties like these, stemming from our current cultural semiotics that privileges machines over experts in terms of objectivity, and biology over social causes in agency. Recognizing this means recognizing that the legibility and meaning of expert images is not easily contained and that the unstable category of demonstrative evidence is at the point of breaking when "mere aids to illustrate testimony" become "an expert's only objective proof."

When one judge decided to minimize the effect of the CT scans in Hinckley's trial, or another judge decided to admit PET evidence but not to allow the jury to see the scans, they were acknowledging some of these consequences, that the images can speak louder than the experts who are and can be their interpreters. The risk is that the images no longer function as mirrors of the scientific process or even of reality but instead as "a binding of fantasies to images and meaning" (de Lauretis 1987, p. 53). These include fantasies of automation without automators, objectivity without the craft and art and messy humanness of scientists, and neutrality without acknowledging the struggles over human categories like normality, mental illness, insanity, and even variability. In short, these digital images risk producing a democracy without people.

PET scanning has appeared in newspapers, popular magazines, and in popular science magazines. To begin considering the role these PET images can play in our own lives, I'd like to reflect for a moment on a stunning article that appeared in the industry magazine, *Advance Radiology* (Hatfield 1995b).

PET Shows Female Brain Has Evolved More Than Male's

The article title itself already presumes a priority of the technology of vision — "PET Shows . . ." The statement is one of fact, of an order in the world revealed by a science and a technology, and the factual order contains categories of significant personal difference (female versus male), a moral hierarchy of personhood (female as more evolved), and a location of personhood (evolution lies in the brain). As I picked up the issue of *Advance* that carried that article title, at a meeting of the Society of Nuclear Medicine, and showed it to different researchers, I found expressions of fascination, surprise, disgust, and humor. "Wild claims are the hallmark of this field," one researcher said to me. "Look here at my poster — I could have written ten pages of conclusions if I had wanted to, but I would have been making it all up!" The article in question has no such constraints:

> Positron emission tomograph (PET) has revealed a major finding: The brains of most men and women are different and women may be slightly more evolved than men.
>
> The study also sheds more light on the theory that human behavior is biologically controlled rather than learned. . . .

Dr. Gur brought up a graph on his computer. The graph charted the differences in metabolic activity in the brains of men and women. Its base is the PET research Dr. Gur had done with his colleagues, including his wife Raquel, a neurologist and psychiatrist.

The graph referred to by Dr. Gur represents a study of 37 male and 24 female, right-handed volunteers who underwent PET. During scanning, which was conducted in a dimly lit room, the subjects were instructed to remain quiet and relaxed, but to try not to close their eyes or fall asleep. Radiolabeled glucose was administered intravenously and each was positioned in a custom-molded head holder during image acquisition.

Glucose metabolism studies also showed that women have more activity in the front area of the brain, which is associated with planning, abstraction and mental flexibility. In this area, men have lower activity and lose brain cells three times as fast as women, he said. That women lose less brain cells and have higher rates of blood flow may suggest why they live longer, Dr. Gur added. Such activity is also prevalent in schizophrenic patients, who have become a prominent part of the Gur's research. (Hatfield 1995b)

First let us note that "men" and "women" are being studied in their statistical sense. Their average metabolism is different, which does not necessarily imply anything about individual men or women. Nonetheless, on the basis of this average difference, Dr. Gur feels free to talk as if the study has implications for how all men and women differ in their daily interactions. Also reporting on the same study by the Gurs, *Newsweek* notes parenthetically that

. . . (the pair got into the field of sex differences when they were struck by their own temperamental differences. He is more intrigued by numbers and details, she likes to work with people; he reacts to a setback by taking a deep breath and moving on, she analyzes it.) (Begley 1995)

Note the circularity wherein the Gurs claim to have taken their own noticed differences as instances or examples of gendered differences: a cultural noticing of a particular kind. Obviously they knew of notions of such differences before, but without attributing significance. At some point, then, they found themselves (one or both) explaining *themselves* via this difference. In other words, idiosyncratic, individual, or personal expressions were reframed as expressions of biological type. The form of the type then remained unknown: Was this due to genotype, phenotype, or chemotype? They therefore were motivated to explore these differences further. For these neuroscientists, it was not enough that

135

gender was an explanation of their social differences; they now wanted a biological explanation of (this kind of) gender. Clearly, it must be pointed out, they were not going to be disappointed. We can safely imagine that if their experiment did not display any significant differences between the men and the women tested, they would *not* have rethought their first gendered explanation of their differences. Rather, they would have assumed that their machines had not had enough resolution.

"There," he said, moving his finger across the blue-gray image on the computer screen, pointing out where metabolic activity is the same in the brain of both sexes. "And here is where it switches," he said, denoting another area that he called the cingulate gyrus.

The cingulate gyrus, according to Dr. Gur, is located in the "new limbic" part of the brain. Together with the "old limbic," the parts make up the overall limbic system of the brain, where emotion is processed.

As explained by Dr. Gur, women have more metabolic activity in the new limbic area, which is more developed in advanced species, such as monkeys. Men, he said, have more metabolic activity in the old limbic area, which controls more primitive ways of responsiveness. "The old limbic, also called the temporal-limbic system, is already quite well developed in the brains of reptiles."

So, does this mean that the female brain is more evolved than that in males? "Yes and no," answered Dr. Gur. "The no part is that we both have more activity in the highly evolved part of the brain. So, maybe women are a half a step ahead of men." (Hatfield 1995b)

Look at the bonus, the excess, which comes as a result of this discovery: speculation in the form of an explanation. There is not only simple difference (if difference could ever be simple) between men and women, but hierarchical difference. Cleverly, and clearly whimsically, Gur patched together Paul MacLean's popularized triune theory of the brain with these new findings to conjure a truly oxymoronic "fact" (might we say factoid?) — "women are more evolved than men."[9] Gur stated this as if evolution is a quantity (for MacLean and most biologists, mammals evolved "later" than reptiles but are not therefore "more" evolved, because evolution is about fitness within a particular environment) and as if women and men are two different species, so absolutely different as to be on separate evolutionary tracks.

Philosopher David Hull, in examining the concept of "biological species," has noted that it connotes natural kinds, which are "eternal, immutable, and discrete," even though for evolutionary biologists they are none of these. Clearly, the Gurs are researchers who relish playing with popular connotations. Ironically, their previous work found handedness to have significant and even stronger regional activation effects (Gur et al. 1982; Reivich and Alavi 1985). By the logic of the above arguments, left-handers should be viewed as a biological group different and potentially more or less evolved than right-handers.

Let us skip over the further wild speculation on the meaning of the discovered differences, remembering that the experiment had no hypotheses regarding specific areas to begin with and ostensibly was able to discover *that* the two groups were different. The end of this article reveals the biggest surprise. Within this data set that proves the difference between men and women, there are "outliers," men who do not look like the other men, women who do not look like the other women.

> Of his most recent study, Dr. Gur said the patterns of activity were reversed in two of the women and 12 of the men. This, he said, may have a correlation with findings of a new study out of the University of Chicago, called *Sex in America: A Definitive Study*,[10] which is available in book form from Little, Brown and Co. The study suggests that there are twice as many gay men as women in the nation.
>
> "This explains why there are more men that show the female pattern," he said. Referring to the dozen male volunteers which showed activity in the brain that was similar to females, Dr. Gur said: "Conceivably, these men could be homosexual."
>
> Such findings would contradict the belief that homosexuality is a result of one's environment. "Some people think sex differences are entirely environmental," he said. "They become really upset when they are shown differences in the way brains behave. They say it can't be." (Hatfield 1995b)

Out of thirty-seven men, twenty-five (or 68 percent) looked identical enough to be called a type, and twelve (or 32 percent) did not look anything like them. These twelve in fact looked like the majority female type. (How did they look like the majority women? Exactly? Statistically significant? Does it really matter, at this point, to us, or Dr. Gur?) The conclusion from this appears so beyond sense and dignity that readers can only laugh very nervously. Perhaps, Dr. Gur replies, clearly not having asked them, these twelve men are gay. Presumably, the other twenty-five are heterosexual (again, a presumption made without the men having been asked). The twelve would be gay, then, not because of sexual preference or orientation, but because of a feminine brain pattern? Homosexuality here returns to a historically aberrant definition as mechanical inversion (Fausto-Sterling 2000).

The *Newsweek* story treats the same data as a significant problem for drawing any conclusions at all from the study. "Not even the researchers are sure what this means. For one thing, 13 men and four women showed activity more like the other sex" (Begley 1995)[11] Depending on one's position, then, this research is either fascinating or abhorrent, promising or abusive, or simply and troublingly silly.

The ease with which we all learn to "see" these oddly shaped images as photolike pictures of the brain derives from an implicit faith in penetrative powers of X-rays and in technological reproduction.[12] The Gurs seem caught up with the possibility of "really" knowing who we are through the miraculous agency of these new digital prosthetics of vision. These articles, and others published by and about the Gurs, are interventions into the facts of PET and the facts of personhood (Gur et al. 1995; Gur et al. 1994). For PET they provide a thumbnail sketch of diagnostic and speculative power. With regard to personhood, they reify and circumscribe types of humans and relations of cause and effect. Reading these articles, one confronts these facts and is drawn into the virtual community of PET images.

Chapter 5
Traveling Images, Popularizing Brains

. . . Even if any given terminology is a reflection of reality, by its very nature as a terminology it must be a selection of reality; and to this extent it must function also as a deflection of reality.
(Burke 1966, p. 45)

Normal Encounters

PET images appear as computer-generated, technologically objective scans of particular brains at particular moments. In popular arenas, these brain images are highlighted in frames with very simple, often one-word labels that emphasize differences between the subjects rather than qualify them.[1] The frame of PET images in Plate 2 is from a *Newsweek* article on mapping the brain (Begley 1992). In a box are three pairs of images, which the captions describe as brains of specific persons—for example, "The brain of a clinically depressed person shows less activity (right) than that of a healthy person." These captions and the labels, however, transform these individual persons into types of humans: *novice, practiced, depressed, healthy, retarded,* and, above all, *normal*. As readers, we are faced with pairs of markedly different images and labels that tell us that these brain scans show us that these persons are significantly different in their brains. More than that, because these are pictures of their brains and the labels are about mental life, the two together purport to demonstrate how and why these types of people are different kinds of humans.

Having looked at many articles in *Newsweek* and other mass-media magazines, I had decided that the articles were written precisely to capitalize on the potent transparency and familiarity of these images of difference. Surprisingly to me, the editor of the *Newsweek* article, Sharon Begley, did not share my conclusion, nor my analysis. Echoing the PET researchers, Begley estimates that the text of the story compensates for the immediacy of the scans. She is as aware of the dangers of scan-likeness as the researchers she interviews, and like them, she emphasizes her point with visual clarity over complexity:

DUMIT: From the illustration, the "PETting the brain" box, the implication I see is that if not now, then soon, PET will be able to tell us the difference between different kinds of people.

BEGLEY: Well, I don't know. Maybe that is an inference that people drew. That implication was not intentional. I think we are looking at a microcosm. The point was to take known cases; in other words, these were not diagnostic or predictive. These were: you identify the two poles going in, and then you take PET scans of these people. And then you can, lo and behold, see differences. Which is not to say, that if you PET scan the brains of a hundred people walking outside this door, that you can get something as striking, or that these hundred people will fall into these two separate groups. The diagnostic possibilities of PET are something that I didn't address, because I don't think that they are really there. And I really dislike erecting a straw man and knocking him down. I'd rather just not open that subject at all. I think it is silly wasting space that way.

DUMIT: Yes. That is, however, the first thing that jumps to people's head when I show them these. Or an instant critical reaction: "These pictures can't really show that. Why does it look like they can?"

BEGLEY: Well, see, in this case they could, but that is because the diagnosis had been made by other criteria beforehand. Again, the only point was—whatever you have, a mentally retarded person or a schizophrenic, and then a non-whatever, then you can see differences. Which is not to say that in all cases you can. I mean you will get false positives and false negatives.

Chapter 4 established how courts assume the task of identifying abnormality through brain technologies. They did this through the notion of "expert images" that promote difference and type. This chapter looks at how brain images travel many places beyond courtrooms, and how their persuasive power and objective authority over human nature is used in many arenas — science journalism, movies, criminality, mental illness, patient activism, doctors' offices. Each of these arenas is invested with specific notions of "normal" and "abnormal," and running through each of these are the manifest assumptions: *mind = brain*, brains have types, these types are people. These assumptions make up the grounds of truth, or *topoi*. Each of the three locations corresponds to a point of view that make different uses of this same "truth" in different ways. In the popular press — through hope, hype, stigma, and play — a "normal observer" who is also a "good citizen" is situated. Within expert culture, attempts are made to control abnormality through prediction, surveillance, and intervention. Finally, the subjects of brain images — patients — inhabit types, living with abnormality. Their point of view is of an abnormal observer, specifically different from the normal.

Because "none of us really come as strangers to the brain, since the foundational metaphors of brain science pervade popular culture, and have for some time" (Star 1992, p. 205), news and journalism can help shape our notions of "accepted medical knowledge" and even our categories of the patient as person.[2] In the rest of this chapter, I follow this shaping process, examining how facts travel in the world, but also how they never travel alone. Instead they are packaged in the form of stories, explanations, and experiences; as authorized or unauthorized; and as facts, which include definitions of human nature.

Two important questions arise for me, one intellectual and one personal. The first is: What is the status of these facts proclaimed in print under expert technological and scientific authority? This question asks about the difficult unevenness of knowledge in the world: How is it produced and verified, and how does it reach me?

The second question is: What if they are true? This question trips me up, catches me off guard, posing a sublime moment of reflection: What do I believe (what do I know) about mental illness, sexual difference, sexuality difference, my own cognitive abilities, brain patterns, and identity? I am fascinated and horrified by the *possibility* posed here, of a world in which technology can tell me who I truly am. An article on Ruben Gur's work with schizophrenia is headlined "PET may someday help screen for criminal behavior, says PhD" (Hatfield 1995a). It presents a world in which technology can tell who is responsible or sane or rational, and who is not. This article presents "a view of the world that might well be different" from my current one (Martin 1987). Some researchers call this ability "biotechnopower": the attribution to technologies of measurement the authority to decide to which categories we essentially belong (Foucault 1978; Haraway 1991; Rabinow 1992). Thus, like Emily Martin, I find myself stumbling "over accepting [these]

141

scientific medical statements as truth" (Martin 1987, p. 10). The question of the mass media reframes the question of truth, however, calling for an examination of the ways in which "new facts" and new worlds and people are produced, distributed, and incorporated.

Toward a Semiotics of Popular Brain Images

> One obvious solution to the floods of data is to rely on images, whose spatial dimensions, shadings, and color codings can easily express large amounts of data . . . yet in spite of their attractions, or perhaps because of them, images create dangers for both clinicians and researchers—dangers intimately entwined with the benefits that imaging technologies confer. One such benefit is the illusion of familiarity. Unlike a table or a chart or graph, an image often seems to be "transparent," giving us the depicted object directly rather than through the mediation of fallible instruments that incorporate certain types of information and leave out others—perhaps equally important—kinds of data. An image can delude us into thinking we know an object in a way a graph never can.
> (Crease 1993, p. 561)

This relationship between image and text is a direct structural reversal of their relationship in the scientific practice described by every researcher with whom I talked, where images were chosen to elaborate textual and quantitative proof. An analogy would be the way in which graphs illustrate textual arguments in scientific articles but are often the sole argument presented in newspaper articles.[3]

Images in texts speak through their captions, which constrain their interpretation. The relationship between image and text in this context is far from simple, however. Historically, according to semiologist Roland Barthes, text represents the authoritative voice behind the jumbled or incomplete appearance of the visible form, structuring perception, telling you how to attend to it, what to attend to in it, and so on. Text does this by reinvigorating the information of the picture: Even if pictures look the same, the text tells you how it is different and why it is worthwhile to look at (Barthes 1983). Barthes points out how in fashion magazines, the reader needs the text to explain *how* to appreciate the value of the newest style. In examining the role of press photos, however, Barthes performed a contrary analysis, proposing that in some cases, the image overtakes the text, overturning the authority of the text. Here the picture provides the compelling anchor:

> The text constitutes a parasitic message intended to connote the image, i.e., to "enliven" it with one or more secondary signifieds. In other words, and this is an important historical reversal, the image no longer illustrates the words; it is the words which, structurally, are parasitic on the image. This reversal has its price: in the traditional modes of "illustration," the image used to function as an episodic return denotation, starting from a principal message (the text), which was perceived as connoted, precisely because it needed an illustration; in the present relation, the image does not come to illuminate or "re-alize" the words; it is the words which come to sublimate, patheti-cize, or rationalize the image. (Barthes 1988, p. 14)

Extending Barthes's argument, this chapter proposes that scientific vi-sualizations, such as PET images, participate in this reversal of veridictory authority. They do so especially when they leave the close community of researchers who daily deal with their semiotic complexity and are aware of their illustrative rather than veridictory use in scientific presentations. Outside of this community, I am interested in how PET images can sometimes become the central argument, with the text as supplement. In the popular arena, in magazines, newspapers and on television, PET images become the principle message. The images and their immediate labels stand as proof, which is then elaborated in textual commentary.

This aspect of analysis focuses on the constellation of codes of "ob-jectivity," "normality," "automaticity," and "veracity" at work within these images. In other words, this strategy tracks the ways in which we learn to see, and learn to believe in seeing. This is a combination of cultural studies, anthropology, and semiotics at the heart of much recent work in cultural studies and feminist studies of science—historical and social. This work draws much inspiration from that of Donna Haraway, Evelyn Fox Keller, Barbara Stafford, and Susan Leigh Star. These schol-ars wade into the tropics of discourse in order to locate and analyze ongoing struggles over the fabric of meaning.

Viewed as signs, PET images in popular culture raise questions of reference and representation—producing the world they are produced by and are part of. They may, building the analysis of the previous chapter, be analyzed within semiotics.

> The project of semiotics should be such mapping [of the discon-tinuity between discourse and reality]: how the physical properties of bodies are socially assumed as signs, as vehicles for social meanings,

and how these signs are culturally generated by codes and subject to historical modes of sign production. (de Lauretis 1984, p. 25)

As discussed in chapter 4, seeing a multicolored blob as a brain image is the result of a learning to see. Semiotically, the familiarity engendered by images of the brain cannot be *simply* apprehended. After all, very few people have ever seen a brain, much less a slice of a brain. Yet, as Ian Hacking has argued, "likeness" — the similarity of one thing to another — can stand alone. Looking at an artifact recovered from an archaeological dig, Hacking noted that though he did not have any idea what was is supposed to be like, he nevertheless knew that it *was* a likeness of something — it was a figure (Hacking 1983). Are PET scans likenesses in the same way?[4] Do we see an image as "like a brain"? For whom are they likenesses?

Ernst Gombrich (1973) has developed a more processual description in which the perceived similarity between the actual referent and the image is more the result of the *process* by which we interpret both of them than of any correspondence between the two. Anne Barry (1997) elaborated this further, noting that we "pick out concepts from the image" like we do from the world. Learning to see forms results in a "meaningful image that contains a story" (p. 139). Barry's insight was that even if perceiving an image is primary to, or does not even need, its caption, it nonetheless is always a contextual, narrated practice, drawing on and drawing together concepts:

> To perceive the world, to grasp the meaning of a drawing, and to create a satirical image: each of these depends on the grasp of essential characteristics and the implications of these as symbolic — that is, as they suggest relationships or tell a story. (Barry 1997, p. 79)[5]

Brain images are powerful, memorable condensers of cultural content and concepts of human nature in this manner. Two adjacent images that look different ask to be seen as the essential characteristics of the labels that describe them. Philosopher Nelson Goodman provided an excellent description of two kinds of classification work taking place with these images (Goodman 1973; Star 1992). On the one hand, there is the assignment of people to presumably preexisting groups: This person is placed in the category "normal" and that person into "depressed." On the other hand, different kinds of groups are being defined on the basis of relations of mutual difference: Normal people are shown to share a characteristic that is different from those of depressed people. Reading the accompanying text reveals a heroic story of the technological quest to produce a beautiful and interpretable image of the brain in action, a quest that is in the process of being fulfilled. I am interested in the fact that it is quite difficult to look at these framed images and not be caught up with the possibility of showing, once and for all, neutrally and objectively, the true difference between these "types" of persons.

Being "caught" refers to the anthropological analyses of Jeanne Favret-Saada (1980), Susan Harding (1987, 1991), and Lorraine Kenny (Kenny 1992). In examining witchcraft, fundamentalist Christianity, and middle-class female adolescence, respectively, these ethnographers watched themselves and others face situations that are initially alien but that draw on existing inclinations, desires, and other cultural aspects of their personhood to draw them into a new viewpoint. Being "caught" means finding yourself wondering just how true some fundamental claim about the world and yourself might be—it means being on the fence, undecided but tipping toward a worldview that is not quite yours . . . yet. In Susan Harding's term, drawn from the language of evangelical faith, it means being "under conviction."[6]

Being "caught" by a brain image is a particular form of identification. In its popular usage, a brain image is akin to the simplified reality of a graphic cartoon, which Scott McCloud (1993), in his fascinating analysis, *Understanding Comics: The Invisible Art*, has described as "a form of amplification through simplification that focuses our attention on an idea" (pp. 30–31). McCloud pays particular attention to the manner in which cartoon drawings achieve indentification:

> Just as our awareness of biological selves are simplified conceptual images—so too is our awareness of these extensions [to cars, clothing, tools] greatly simplified. . . . Our identities belong permanently to the conceptual world. They can't be seen, heard, smelled, touched or tasted. They're merely ideas and everything else—at the start—belongs to the sensual world, the world beyond us. . . . By de-emphasizing the appearances of the physical world in favor of the idea of form, the cartoon places itself in the world of concepts. . . . When cartoons are used through a story, the world of that story may seem to *pulse with life*. (pp. 39–41)

Our identity, as biological, as personalities, and in relationships, is here shown open to conceptual revision. Cartoon are especially good, McCloud has suggested, at inviting one to inhabit them:

> When you look at a photo or realistic drawing of a face—you see it as the face of *another*. But when you enter the world of the cartoon—you see *yourself*. . . . The cartoon is a vacuum into which our identity and awareness are pulled . . . an empty shell that we inhabit which enables us to travel in another realm. We don't just observe the cartoon, we *become* it! (p. 36)

145

Cartoons or other abstract images, amplified through simplification like brain images are, provide a conceptual bridge, a connecting self, a human nature, and a set of categories. The difference between a fictional cartoon and a brain image is that the realm of the latter is science, and its concepts thus subtend rather than extend our everyday identification.

An example of a brain-difference fact may help emphasize this confrontation between a reader and a brain image. In an editorial in *U.S. News & World Report* entitled "Sex: It's All in Your Brain," writer John Leo launched into a diatribe against those who have "a curious refusal, based on politics, in spite of a large body of evidence," to acknowledge that men and women just *are* biologically, and hence socially, different. Citing a front-page story in the *New York Times* on functional magnetic resonance, he wrote:[7]

> The photo that ran with last week's study may help break down this resistance. It's a magnetic resonance image of a male brain and a female brain attempting the same task — sounding out words. The image — apparently the first graphic, visual proof of difference in the brains — shows that the male used only a small part of the left side of the brain, while the female used both sides. . . . Some scientists think this may help explain the male's famous inability to express emotion: Information flows less easily from the right side to the verbal, left side. (Leo 1995)

Although Leo seemed to think the article clarified the issue, many issues must be unpacked in this media intervention. The article mediates between experts who presumably provided the details of brains and brain images and us layperson viewers.[8] Though some might want to claim that there is a set of accepted medical truths (and unfortunately that there are some unacceptable lies that get taken up), the purpose of this chapter and this book is to work with a notion of uneven flows of knowledge and contradictory versions of acceptability and legitimacy. As laypersons, we do not know how much we do not know about scientific and medical truths, yet we, like Leo, are caught up in the possibility of explaining ourselves through them.

McCloud provided a useful summary of the semiotic process through which cartoons — and, by extension brain images — in popular culture work (McCloud 1993, p. 46):

Complex   →   Simple
Realistic   →   Iconic
Objective   →   Subjective
Specific   →   Universal

The key point for brain imaging is that as the image becomes more simple and iconic, it also becomes more subjective (personally invested in) and universal (generalizable to human nature). I suggest that these neuroscienctific facts compel such reworking because they provide authoritative starting points along with combinatory possibilities. Like Levi-Strauss's totem animals and Turkle's computers, they are good and solid and fun to think with, lively facts with provocative connotations (Levi-Strauss 1963; Turkle 1984).[9]

Expert Selves, Anxious Measures

> The logic was straightforward. Behind every thought or feeling, there was a molecular reaction in the brain. Behind every molecule in the reaction, there was an enzyme that created the molecule; behind every enzyme was a gene.
>
> If the gene was defective, the enzyme would be defective; if the enzyme was defective, so would be the molecule; if the molecule was defective, so would be the chemical reaction and so, inevitably, would be the thought the reaction produced. Or, as one scientist simplified it, in a few words with many levels of meaning, "Twisted molecules lead to twisted thoughts."
>
> (Franklin 1987, p. 146)

The rhetorical image of the brain as viewed by the social expert is one of anxiety. The normal brain is taken as a baseline of social norms, but if the brain is perturbed, it goes only one way, down, into abnormality, into personal and social problems. In this world of constant brain risk, the job of the brave new science of molecular psychology is to predict, surveil, and intervene whenever brains deviate.

> Aggressive behavior seems to be built into human genes, and is encouraged daily by environmental forces. Linked to that aggression is fear. Both emotions are thought to be reflected in measurable changes in the chemistry of the brain. . . .
>
> During the 1960s and 70s, attention shifted toward socioeconomic factors, such as poverty and lack of education, as important contributors to aggressiveness or criminal behavior. Today the pendulum swings back and forth in the nurture vs. nature debate as more new information is brought to light. The question remains whether environment or heredity is the main cause of aggressive human behavior. With PET imaging, we can begin to explore the degree to which biological and social factors affect brain chemistry. Perhaps one day we

will speak of an individual's brain chemotype as well as his or her genotype and phenotype. (Wagner and Ketchum 1989, pp. 171–172).

Metaphors, narratives, and explanations abound as to what the brain is, how it works, and its implications for our minds and the minds of others. Lived metaphors — embodied in documents and technologies — are here treated as the contestable terrain of the social world. These methods foreground the processes by which categories and relationships such as objectivity and normality are produced and maintained.[10] Wagner said, in an interview:

> My present research with PET scanning is concerned with investigating chemical reactions constantly taking place inside the human brain, and how these reactions affect how we think, feel and act . . . how they affect whether we are afraid, violent or destructive. . . . Perhaps we will be able to learn enough about the brain chemistry of fear, violence, and destructiveness to save ourselves from the problems of interpersonal violence and war.

Built into Wagner's approach to the brain is a notion of human nature in which violence is the product of brain chemistry.[11] Other notions of human nature, whether drawn from capitalism, patriarchy, or religion, point to violence as socially and/or morally caused. Wagner's notion of violence and destructiveness also presumes a particular configuration and explanation of rationality. Rational violence, or even violence as a rational response to social conditions, is probably oxymoronic.[12] In his view, violence is bad, violence is destructive, and violence is irrational.[13] Before I get carried away, however, I want to note that there are many compelling facts and reasons to assume and act on this notion of human nature.[14] My point here is to flag the powerful explanatory consequences accompanying experiments on the brain.

Your Brain on Ecstasy

Four kinds of escalating rhetoric describe the same study of MDMA (3,4-methylenedioxy methamphetamine, or ecstasy) users. In 1998, a PET study was done of 14 people who used MDMA heavily compared with 15 nonusers. The results were significant both mathematically and socially. The study concluded:

> . . . these data suggest that human MDMA users are susceptible to MDMA-induced brain 5-HT neural injury. . . . Our data do not allow conclusions about reversibility or permanence of MDMA-induced changes in brain 5-HT transporter. (McCann et al. 1998)

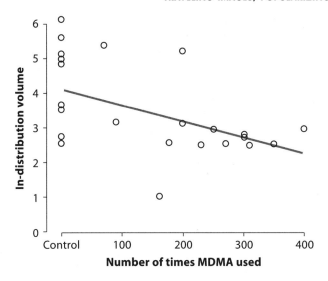

FIGURE 5.1. Ecstasy user's brain graph. (From McCann, Szabo, Scheffel, et al. 1998)

Its publication in *Lancet* was followed by the appearance of a series of letters calling into question the parameters and generalizability of the study. Included in the article was a series of scans, charts, and graphs illustrating how the range of neurotransmitter activity differed among the two groups. Among other problems, the range overlapped so much that if the data were in fact generalizable, one might be able to make a guess but certainly not a diagnosis of someone's past drug use on the basis of a scan (figure 5.1). Nonetheless, the images published with the study were of one individual from each group, each looking extremely different. It appeared as if they were, in fact, the extremes (see Plate 16).

As the study results traveled outside of the medical journal, the stated implications intensified. In the newsletter *NIDA Notes*, staff writer Robert Mathias described the broad outline of the study and discussed the overall results in a competent manner as a correlation.[15] In the caption to the image included with the article, though, he claimed it showed causality: "Dark areas in the MDMA user's brain show damage due to chronic MDMA use."

When the images traveled to the U.S. Senate Caucus on International Narcotics Control, however, the director of the National Institute on Drug Abuse (NIDA) used them to proclaim not only absolute causality but diagnostic ability as well: "Through the use of positron emission

149

tomography (PET), we can actually see that the brain images on top belongs to an individual who has never used MDMA. . . . Clearly the brain of the MDMA user on the bottom has been significantly altered."[16]

At this point, the extreme images of two people were being used to ground a strong biosocial claim, not to illustrate a weak one, as they did in the *Lancet* article. It should come as no surprise, then, that the NIDA 25-year poster took the further step of creating a single didactic image about the ecstasy brain images (see Plate 17).

Building on the "your brain on drugs" campaign, this poster visually argued that twisted drugs lead to twisted brains (and therefore to a twisted self). The poster also went a step too far. As if the choosing of color scales, windowing ranges, and extreme images is not enough, in combining the right half of a "normal brain" with the left half of a "brain on ecstasy," the graphic artists actually inverted the color scale of purple and black. The result is an even more stunning and tragic looking drug-ravaged brain, but at the expense of putting forth a visual lie.

Images of *Rampage*

Considering the role these images can play in our own lives from a different angle, the following is an example of PET as depicted in a popular film about schizophrenia, violence, and insanity. What follows is my transcript of the final four minutes of *Rampage* (1988), directed by William Friedkin. I believe it represents the first use of PET in a Hollywood movie. At this point in the film, Charles Reese has committed six grisly murders and is about to be found guilty of them by a jury.

> *In a courtroom.*
> DEFENSE ATTORNEY: [*whispering to his client, Charles Reese, just convicted of six brutal first-degree (premeditated) murders*] We still have a shot to save your life. We can still show the jury that you weren't responsible.
> *Cut to the judge's chamber.*
> DEFENSE ATTORNEY: Your honor, I'm going to request that a PET scan be performed as part of a defense to show the jury that he is mentally ill, during the penalty phase.
> PROSECUTOR: A PET scan purports to show only a patient's brain chemistry at a certain moment of time. In this case it is after the crime is committed.
> JUDGE: A PET scan is a form of medical imaging which is used in the diagnosis of epilepsy, some Alzheimer's, as well as mental deficiency. Depriving Mr. Reese of putting this in front of the jury—

150

PROSECUTOR: [*interrupting*] It's only another gadget to hide Mr. Reese's responsibility.

JUDGE: [*pausing, contemplating*] Well, we're going to err on the side of caution. I'm going to order the test. We'll let the jury evaluate it. Nobody knows what it will show.

> *Cut to medical laboratory. Charles Reese is put in the PET scanner. A rotating skull is shown, computer generated, peeling back to reveal a rotating brain in red, then green.*

> *Two scans come up side by side. One says "Normal Control" under it; the other says "Reese, Charles." The scans look very visibly different.*

MEDICAL DOCTOR: [*pointing to Reese's scan*] These are abnormal patterns without a doubt.

DEFENSE ATTORNEY: What does that tell you?

MEDICAL DOCTOR: Well, this yellow-green area here is consistent with schizophrenia. What you are seeing is a computer-enhanced image of the chemistry of the brain. And what it shows is a picture of madness.

> *Cut to the courtroom again.*

JURY FOREMAN: Your honor, based on the new scientific evidence, we, the jury, find that the defendant should go to a state mental hospital.

> *At the end of the movie, words: "Charles Reese has served four years in a state mental facility. He has had one hearing to determine his eligibility for release. His next hearing is in four months."*

In the microcosm of this movie, a convicted brutal murderer is not put into prison but is treated as a mentally diseased subject who may be released in the near future. The sole element presented to account for the jury's decision is a PET scan.[17] The words of the doctor — "these are abnormal patterns without a doubt . . . consistent with schizophrenia . . . a picture of madness" — concatenate a history of struggle and controversy within the medical and legal communities regarding a host of relationships: PET scan to brain, brain to schizophrenia, schizophrenia to insanity. In the movie, the PET scan stands as the fact, the linchpin referent, that holds the chain of connections together, convincing a jury that an abnormal brain scan is an abnormal brain is an abnormal person who does not bear responsibility for murder.

Not one of these connections, however, is settled in the scientific and medical community, in the legal community, or in my own mind.[18] Medical anthropologist Horacio Fabrega has discussed the reluctance of Anglo-American society to accept a theory of illness-caused deviance. He suggests that this is primarily due to a need to have the will be socially or rationally motivated: "In essence, mental illness as a defense of homicide requires a suspension of our attribution of personhood if the latter is equated with willful symbolic behavior" (Fabrega 1989, p. 592). Although I think that this argument makes sense in general when comparing societies, I am interested in the ways in which the attributes of personhood in the United States are continually contested using batteries of facts. *Rampage* is an intervention into the facts of PET and the facts of life, presenting as it does a definition of PET, a set of presumptions about imaging and mental illness, and a possible scenario of PET's use in a court. As with reading a magazine article on brain imaging, in watching the movie one is faced with facts about one's objective self.[19]

Faced with novel facts in this movie, we may indeed stumble over accepting them. Hollywood movies, along with best-selling novels written by physicians and our own doctors' advice, help to shape our notions of "accepted medical knowledge" and thus help shape our categories of the person.

When I have shown the movie clip from *Rampage* and pictures of PET scans during talks, some people with social constructionist tendencies and some with strong feelings about the social or psychodynamic nature of schizophrenia have been upset over the biosocial totalitarian implications of this apparently seamless presentation of clear difference between "them" and "us." I want first to note that despite constant work on PET and schizophrenia since the 1980s, there is still much disagreement over whether PET is ready yet for clinical work with mental illness. As discussed in chapter 4, most of the PET community furiously opposes the use of PET for the insanity defense. In spite of this unreliability for regular clinical work, in some places PET has nevertheless been heavily supported, including financially, by mental-illness activists, that is, organized families of people with mental illness. Here another set of contests emerges. Should researchers look for biological correlates of schizophrenia, and how should such correlates be interpreted? What do the facts mean? Surprisingly, the meaning of these facts does not emerge solely from the research community; the whole virtual community must be examined.

In the late 1970s and into the 1980s the increasing availability of new diagnostic techniques such as CT and PET scanning contributed greatly to the notion of mental illness as a biological disease or defect. These techniques offered different and exciting ways of examining living brains (Pardes and Pincus 1985). Early on, it was realized that many head injuries, strokes, and epilepsies leave the structure of the brain relatively unchanged but show up with different degrees of clarity on PET scans. In biological psychiatry, such proof of pathology is talked about as a "holy grail." One biological psychiatrist, for instance, began a review of PET with the statement "In the 1970s, the antipsychiatry movement almost had us . . . , but now we have proof" (Kuhar 1989). For this subdiscipline, eager to demonstrate the physiology of mental illness, images of brain differences between mentally ill patients and non — mentally ill control subjects were facts that implied that a full biological explanation of mental disease was only a matter of time.

> Much optimism has been generated in those who feel that the only reason organic bases for the various psychiatric syndromes have not been elucidated has been the lack of a suitable investigative tool. . . . It is probable that PET is the investigative technique of choice for research of such hypotheses in man. (Frackowiak 1986)

Early PET thus functioned as a promise that mental illness was not "in the head" but in the brain. The medical imaging advantage was measured in two ways. First, it allowed correlation between brains and diagnosis among living humans, thus permitting anew the equation of *brain = illness*. Second, medical imaging promised to provide early warnings of the onset of mental illness, one of the largest problems in its treatment and prevention.

Selling PET

The positive side of the expert image in popular culture is the promise of understanding and future cure. This, too, is mediated by anxiety, however.

To illustrate the ongoing negotiation of personhood and illness and call attention to the wider virtual community of objective self-fashioning around PET, I turn now to one site of my fieldwork, the Brain Imaging Center at the University of California, Irvine. This center was unlike most PET centers in two important respects. First, it was located in a psychiatry department, not in a chemistry, nuclear medicine, or radiology department. Second, for a PET center, it was extremely underfunded. Other major PET centers have received either Department of Energy or National Institutes of Health program grants to support the multimillion-dollar costs of laboratories in nuclear medicine or radiology. This center's program, in constrast, was started in a psychiatry department, and the scanner and cyclotron were purchased with bank loans. Monthly payments were dependent on an external fee schedule that dampened free operation. In the words of one researcher, Dr. Joseph Wu, a psychiatrist at the University of California, Irvine:

> I think we were sort of an upstart . . . because other places that have PET centers are much better endowed than we were. We were

sort of the scrappy, come-from-behind, shoestring budget kind of guys. And we did things on a budget that is probably one-tenth of the budget that Hopkins [and] UCLA [have] for their PET centers. They are very well endowed and they support their PET centers in a maximum way. I think that we have a much more sort of guerrilla-type operation. We are unconventional in that we did so many things on our own, but I think we were fairly productive.

This PET center operated from such a precarious financial position that its researchers spent much time doing local community outreach, and they found a ready alliance with the mental-illness community in Orange County, especially with families who had schizophrenic children. As Haier detailed below, the psychodynamic approach, while supporting the social nature of schizophrenia, often localized this causation in the family and, more specifically, in the mother.

[One family] contributed $250,000 to help pay for our scanner. By that time, the scanner had arrived and we were making pictures. They had schizophrenia in their family, and they were very interested in it. They knew our emphasis was going to be on schizophrenia. We always approach it that in the long run, the main help will come through research. Probably not for people who currently have it, but because there is a genetic component, there are still the grandchildren to worry about. And families find this compelling. Remember, even in the late '80s, the public was just coming out of the idea of the schizogenic mother, that schizophrenia was somehow induced because the mother was doing something wrong. Virtually every set of parents that we talk to now, when schizophrenics are now in their twenties and their thirties, almost every parent has had the experience of going to a psychologist early on and getting the idea that somehow they were at fault. So it is all in their memory. And the idea that it is biological has caught on real fast over the last five or eight years. Family groups have organized around this to support biological research, and imaging is obviously at the heart of that. So it is kind of a natural sequence of events.

Supporting PET research became a means for these families to empower their participation within science, stay informed, and come to understand their role as accountable to, but not responsible for, the fact of familial schizophrenia. Along with the National Alliance for the Mentally Ill (NAMI), these families advocated a biological redefinition of mental illness and actively helped to produce facts about the nature of personhood and mental illness (Office of Technology Assessment 1992). Objective self-fashioning here is a strategy without which such research might not get done.

Using PET to Sell

> Identifying brain activity associated with depression and the changes that result from treatment and the patient's improved mood will help to destigmatize the illness, a disease of the brain.
> —National Institute of Mental Health Web site

There is yet another purpose for PET scans in contemporary biomedical America: public relations. The power of brain images to directly interpolate their viewers is often explicitly used as a technique of persuasion. Almost all of the mental disorders on the Web site of the National Institute of Mental Health and in its pamphlets embody the sentiment expressed in the quotation above. Through paired brain images of normal people and of those with disorders, and through images of a treatment's effect on the brain, people may be persuaded that mental illnesses are, in fact, biological. Brain images are here the ground of proof of the claims (see Plate 18).

In an interesting counterpoint, Jeffrey Schwartz used PET images on the back of his self-help book *Brainlock* for obsessive-compulsive disorder to demonstrate/prove that cognitive behavioral therapy can alter the brain as much as drugs. Treatment—whether drugs or psychology—lends itself to images demonstrating cure (see Plate 15).

These paired images of self and possible future self can be understood as participating in the larger topos of "before and after" pictures, as discussed by Dorothy Smith. Smith unpacked the discourse of femininity by focusing in part on fashion images in women's magazines. She notes that these images must be carefully understood within the context of their use; they are embedded within texts that apparently contain descriptions of how to make oneself over, to look and feel and be *better*. In this context, the fashion image works to construct the reader as a "subject" for betterment. The reader becomes an imperfect subject vis-à-vis the ideal one pictured, but one who can potentially become better through remediation. In other words, a diverse array of aesthetic positions are collapsed into two poles, ugly (undesirable) and beautiful (desirable), with the implication that the reader is either the former or the latter.

Smith described how the subject is thus entered into a discursive organization of desire, a desire that exists, she noted, even when the subject has no hope of achieving the ideal. The paradigmatic images in this regard are the "before" and "after" images. "*Before* identifies for the looker the critical state from which to begin to produce the self or other

155

body into the end-state, *after*" (Smith 1990). The "before" and "after" images contain the coordinates of a course of action and between them, a gap, which is desire, created by the negativity of one and the positivity of the other. The positive one becomes the ideal.

Many PET images of abnormal and normal participate (willingly or unwillingly) in this public discourse of before and after. By showing extreme differences between two states, these images appear to collapse a diverse array or continuum of people into two kinds. They simultaneously offer PET as the remedial technology that can clearly make the distinction between these two kinds. In the context of medical scientific images, these differences are transformed not only into the idea of a perfect diagnosis[20] (Stafford 1991) but also into the possibility of a cure (Ginsburg and Rapp 1995). In each of these cases, the PET images work to create the present possibility of differentiating between two states. In the process it also hardens and reifies these states. These verifications also impel action. Visualizations used in this extreme and exemplary fashion thus function as powerfully potent transformers of statistical norms into ideal and abhorred *qualities*.

Toward a Dynamic Category of the Person

> We must learn to distinguish it [the body which I live and experience, just as I live and experience it] from the objective body as set forth in works on physiology. This is not the body which is capable of being inhabited by a consciousness.
> — Merleau-Ponty[21]

Marcel Mauss and others following him argued that the basic human unit, "the person," is a cultural category with different attributes — for example, rationality, agency, participation, gender divisions — for different cultures in different times and places.[22] For Mauss and his successors, the *person* is a category stuffed into a physical body but independent of the body's physicality. They argue as if each culture or historical period has its own category of the person. Other anthropologists have been more troubled by the findings of medicine and neuroscience. For instance, Victor Turner once expressed great difficulty in keeping up with the latest findings: "This is because I am having to submit to question some of the axioms anthropologists . . . were taught to hallow. These axioms express the belief that all human behavior is the result of social conditioning. Clearly a very great deal of it is, but gradually it has been borne home to me that there are inherent resistances to conditioning" (Turner 1983, p. 211). Turner was describing how new facts from medicine and neuroscience disturbed his notion of personhood and personal behavior. Facing these facts requires reimagining what kinds of persons humans are. How do we as anthropologists and other scholars understand our bodies? How do we put together the facts of science and medicine, as we read them in the *New York Times* and receive them from our doctors, with the role of culture in our constitution? In anthropological terms, I am interested in how facts come to play a role in our everyday category of the person.

Medical anthropologists have long faced the relation between what Merleau-Ponty called our objective body and our lived body, or our person, with a variety of more subtle analyses. For clinical medical anthropology, oriented around the question of efficacy, the lived body (cultural) and the objective body (physiology) have initially different causes but mutually influence each other throughout development. For example, physiological diseases are often inseparable from cultural variables such as diet.[23] In spite of this flexibility, each culture is ultimately assigned its "body" that is lived and explained in relation to an objective body, which provides the touchstone of cross-cultural comparison and criticism. *Change* in the category of the person is not well identified. Instead, categories are often explained as a reflection of changes in other spheres of society: economics, politics, colonization, and religion.[24]

Within other medical anthropologies, some sociologies of medicine, and the history of science and medicine, a different approach is taken. Instead of the experience of health and illness as variable, the "objective body" is taken as culturally and historically contingent. The body is understood as the object of a scientific and medical gaze that changes with the times, the discipline, site, culture and circumstance.[25] These approaches understand the objective body to vary with the development (positive or negative) of technoscientific culture, attending to how the historical-cultural category of the person (via politics, economics, etc.) influences the evaluation of the objective body.[26] The objective body and the experienced body remain side by side, both variable but analytically separate.[27]

Is it possible that local mutations in categories of people take place daily, that they are contested within American cultures because they are lived and not just known? The example of the Gurs, and the following example from popular psychiatry, will help to propose a dynamic notion of the category of the person.

In his 1993 nonfiction bestseller, *Listening to Prozac*, the author, psychiatrist Peter Kramer, began with the following story. Kramer was visited by a patient, Sam, who suffered from a brooding depression following the death of his parents. Kramer first prescribed an antidepressant that did not seem to have an effect. Feeling that a different kind of antidepressant might help, Kramer proposed Prozac, which Sam agreed to try.

> The change, when it came, was remarkable: Sam not only recovered from his depression, he declared himself "better than well." He felt unencumbered, more vitally alive, less pessimistic. Now he could complete projects in one draft, whereas before he had sketched and sketched again. His memory was more reliable, his concentration keener. Every aspect of his work went more smoothly. He appeared more poised, more thoughtful, less distracted. . . . Though he enjoyed sex as much as ever, he no longer had any interest in pornography. . . . He experienced this change as a loss. The style he had nurtured and defended for years now seemed not a part of him but an illness. What he had touted as independence of spirit was a biological tic. In particular, Sam was convinced that his interest in pornography had been mere physiological obsessionality. . . . This one aspect of his recovery was disconcerting, because the medication redefined what was essential and what was contingent about his own personality—and the drug agreed with his wife when she was being critical. Sam was under the influence of medication in more ways than one: he had allowed Prozac not only to cure the episode of depression but also to tell him how he was constituted. . . . Though I had never taken psychotherapeutic medication, I, too, seemed to be under its influence. (Kramer 1993, p. xi)

Sam became more alert, attentive, happy, adjusted, and "successful" than ever before in his life. Kramer also saw this about Sam, and realized that both he and his patient then understood the "real" Sam to be the one that Prozac revealed, and the former Sam to be a biological sickness. Sam and Kramer had "listened to Prozac" rather than to Sam's previous three decades of life. Because Prozac is a biological drug, Sam must in some sense have been cured by it, freed at last from his strange psychophysiological disease and able to be his true self, and his true self became something that was perhaps revealed only with Prozac. That Sam took Prozac and then behaved differently (and better), I want to note as a fact-in-the-world, to help keep in mind that facts do not just pop into our consciousness. Facts have to find us, and we have to incorporate them as facts.

Sam's story is not just an anecdote—it is an apparently objective account made as part of a psychiatrist's case history. We know this "fact" about Sam only through the story told by Peter Kramer, M.D. I almost want to call this "fact" a factoid to call attention to the specific ways that we *learn* the fact, that we attend to all of the cultural aspects of our learning: the objective voice, the authorship of a psychiatrist, doctor, scientist, book-writer, the way in which Kramer's discussion of his own disconcertedness and surprise allows us to share these feelings as part of the novelty of this fact.[28] This story is a challenge for us, to deny it or fit it into our categories of people. These are ways in which the story makes sense to us, as possible, even as it pushes our notions of what is possible.

We are the sorts of people who take facts seriously, but *how* do we take them so? How do we incorporate them into ourselves—especially the ones that shape who we are but that we ourselves are not equipped to test? Even if we can test them, the fact also comes along with a contextual delineation of human nature. In other words, is it possible to ask how facts become these sorts of things for us, without getting involved immediately in questions over the truth value of them?

Facts usually imply relationships between things that are not bound to time and space and culture; they simply are. Facts are not untethered, however; facts are facts-in-the-world. My project is to understand how the meaning of facts change—how we are never simply handed the facts but are continually faced with facts-in-the-world and continually judging the status and relative worth of them for ourselves.[29]

Facts are bits of mastery in an expert culture. Expert culture is about being extremely knowledgeable about a very few things. We are all people who know a little about quite a lot of things, but, in their entirety, the facts are beyond reach. The very category of the person has become, in part, parceled out among expert discourses. All facts contain, imply, or exclude categories of people, and calling the case of Sam a fact-in-the-world attempts to mnemonically maintain the perspective that a particular category of the person is at stake in the "fact," and that this fact has traveled.

We must ask ourselves, however, why this Prozac story can be so compelling, and why we consider it authoritative. One objection to the above description might be that Sam *experienced* a new self, and it was so compelling that he simply adopted it as his true self. Kramer and Sam's friends did the same because they *experienced* a different Sam as well. This does not account, however, for my feelings and others' on *hearing* about Sam. In discussing this case, I have been struck by a double response. On the one hand, there is a desire to have it not be true, to deny the fact of the transformation and assert a less mutable category of the person. On the other hand, there is a desire to know more about the stories, to begin to play with the fact and call into question one's own category of the person. My sense is that the fact exploits the incompleteness of our categories of people, that there is much that is either unaccounted for or contradictorily accounted for in

159

our categories, and that each fact provides material "good to think with," in Levi-Strauss's memorable coinage.[30]

What makes *Listening to Prozac* fascinating and recommended reading is that Kramer was well aware of the cultural nature of his understanding of Sam's self, and he was both frightened and eager to work with it. He went on to consider more borderline cases — for instance, a woman who has been "spacy and flaky" all her life. When taking Prozac, she becomes a faster and more articulate speaker. A businessperson taking Prozac becomes less sensitive to all the possible problems in proposals and therefore more risk-taking and successful. These examples raise the dilemma of what Kramer calls "cosmetic psychopharmacology," people who are taking Prozac to become better than their "normal" selves.[31] At stake in these stories are contrasting categories of persons — flakiness and eloquence, risk-taking ability and self-deprecation — as neurochemical on/off switches. These in turn alter how we feel about the drugs: "Once these medicines have colored our view of how the self is constituted, our understanding of related ethical issues inevitably will be affected" (Kramer 1993).

Kramer's work illustrates how at least in the United States, expert scientific and medical *facts* play a key role in how we experience our selves, our bodies, and others. In other words, there appear to be many objective bodies that we inhabit consciously, in part through adjusting our categories of persons to account for compelling facts. Of course this is not a one-way imposition of science on laypeople. Scientific facts affect us, but we are not, as Roger Cooter has pointed out, passive laypeople (Cooter 1984). We participate in the instantiation and legitimation of facts. In the next sections, I consider our role in the business of producing and maintaining facts. For now I want to concentrate on how we incorporate facts into our lived experience.

Embodiment: Facing Brain Facts

The following remarkable passage is from a memoir, *The Beast: A Reckoning with Depression*, written by journalist Tracy Thompson. Extremely depressed, having failed to commit suicide, and in a mental institution, she reacted as follows to a book on the history of depression:

> The idea of depression as a definable illness, documented for millennia, was new [to me.] . . . Depression, then, was a kind of disease, an illness. I'd even said that myself on occasion. But even that had not clarified the confusion; illness was another concept that had layers of meaning. [The first was a real disease with visible effects.]

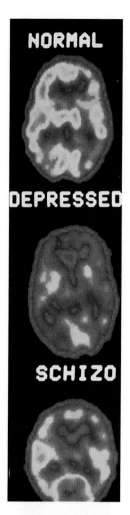

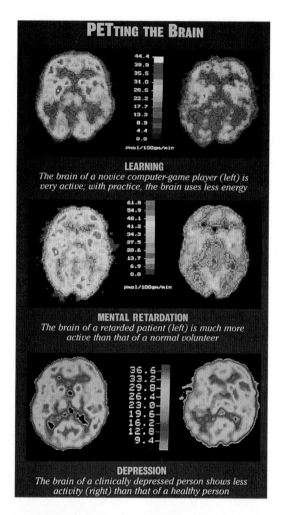

PLATE 1. Positron emissions tomography (PET) scans in *Vogue*; see p. 6 (from "New Seeing-Eye Machines . . . look inside your body, can save your life," by Joseph Hixson, *Vogue*, July 1983)

PLATE 2. PET scans of different functions and traits, in *Newsweek*; see p.139 (from "Mapping the brain (Cover Story)," by Sharon Begley, in *Newsweek* 1992 vol. 66)

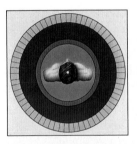

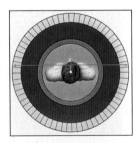

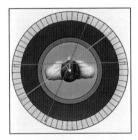

1. Rings of block detectors surround the patient. A single ring on the ECAT is comprised of 512 crystals (8 crystals/detector x 64 detectors).

2. An event is recorded when two crystals detect gamma rays that occur within a coincidence time window. A line of response (LOR) indicates what two crystals detected the event.

3. A unique line of response is identified by the angle and radius of a perpendicular (dashed line) back to the center of the field of view.

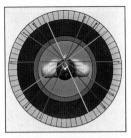

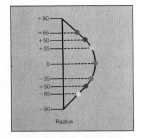

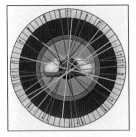

4. As additional events are detected, the lines of response are recorded.

5. Each LOR is plotted using polar coordinates (angle vs. radius). The composite results in a sinusoidal plot of LORs through a single point and is referred to as a sinogram.

6. The multiple LORs through multiple points.

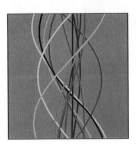

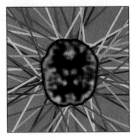

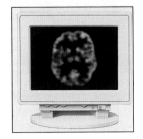

7. The result is a sinogram which is comprised of numerous, overlapping single point plots. The matrix size of the transverse field of view.

8. Following acquistion, filtered back projection algorithms are applied to the sinogram data to produce images.

9. the final image is then ready for display.

PLATE 3. Illustrations of the PET scanning process; see pp. 73, 77 (reproduced with permission from Siemens Medical Solutions USA, Inc.)

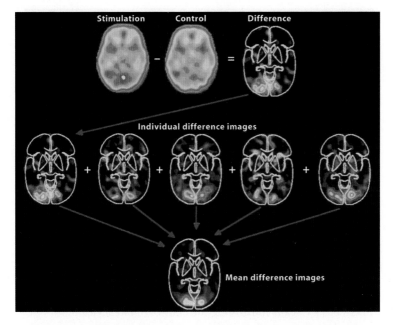

PLATE 4. PET scans illustrating the subtraction and averaging processes; see pp. 86–88 (Posner and Raichle 1994)

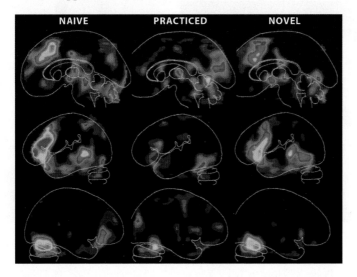

PLATE 5. PET scans of three vertical slices through the brain during a word-generation experiment, illustrating the unpracticed (or naïve) subject, the practiced subject, and the subject performing the task with a novel set of words; see p. 66 (Posner and Raichle 1994)

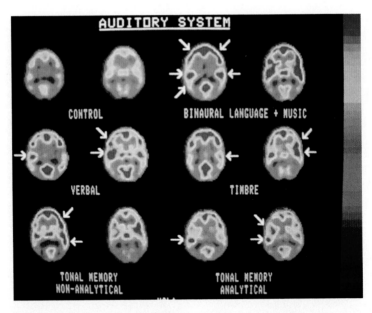

PLATE 6. PET scans illustrating the auditory system; see p.66
(Phelps 1991)

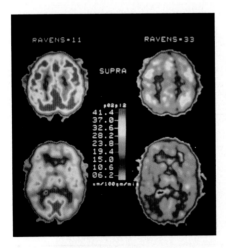

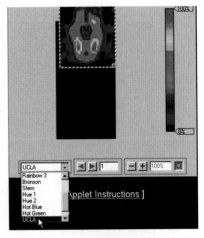

PLATE 7. PET scans of the Ravens Advanced Matrices intelligence test, from Sharon Begley's "How to Tell if You're Smart—See Your Brain Light Up," in *Newsweek* 1988 (vol. 64); see p. 66 (reproduced courtesy of Richard Haier, M.D.)

PLATE 8. Screen capture of the Image Viewer applet (ePET) developed by Val Stambolstian, Ph.D.; see p. 93 (courtesy of the Interactive Media Group, Crump Institute for Molecular Imaging)

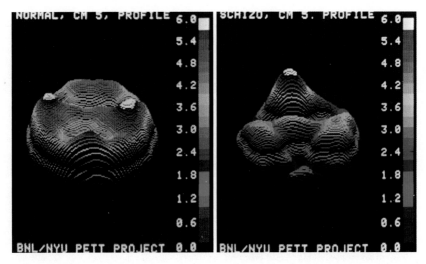

PLATE 9. Three-dimensional PET scans of "normal" and "schizophrenic brains"; see p. 90 (Wolf 1981a; reproduced with permission from Brookhaven National Laboratory)

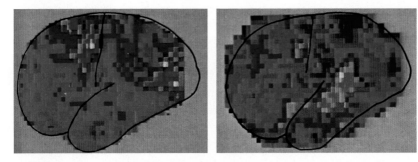

PLATE 10. Xenon blood flow scans; see p. 54 (from Lassen et al. 1970; with permission)

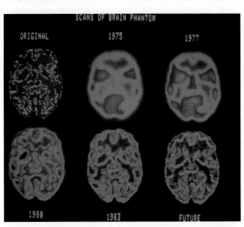

PLATE 11. PET scans of "brain phantoms," showing the evolution of PET scanners at UCLA; see p. 78 (original slide provided by Michael Phelps)

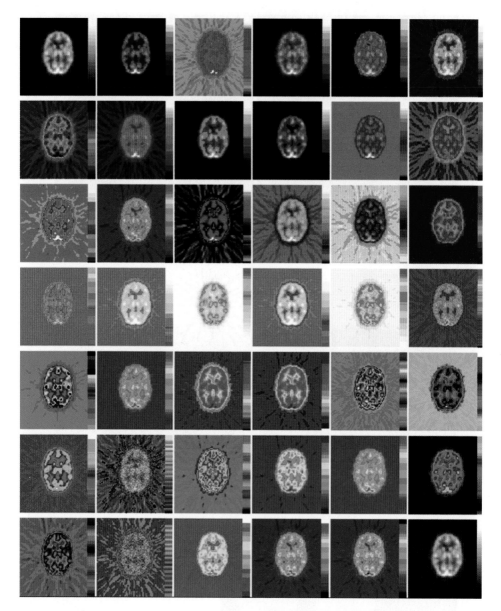

PLATE 12. Identical PET scans illustrating pseudo-color choices; see p. 94 (courtesy of Brian Murphy)

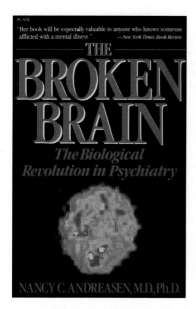

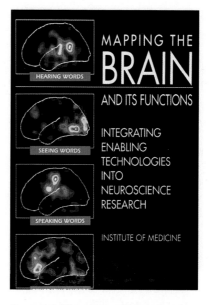

PLATE 13. Paperback cover design for *The Broken Brain*, by Nancy C. Andreasen; see p. 126 (Andreasen 1984)

PLATE 14. The cover of *Mapping the Brain and its Functions*, by Constance Pechura and Joseph Martin; see pp. 19, 88 (Pechura and Marin 1991)

Change your own brain chemistry! Schwartz's groundbreaking studies have shown that by using his Four-Step program you can actually "rewire" your brain and modify your genetic disposition.

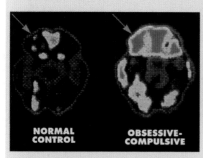

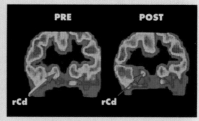

PLATE 15. PET scans of a patient with obsessive-compulsive disorder, showing the brain before and after therapy; from the back cover design of *Brain Lock: Free Yourself from Obsessive-Compulsive Behavior: A Four-Step Self-Treatment Method to Change Your Brain Chemistry*; see p. 155 (courtesy of Jeffrey Schwartz, M.D.)

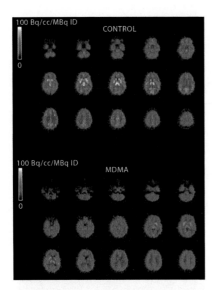

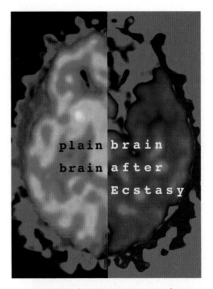

PLATE 16. PET scan of the brain of a heavy user of MDMA ("ecstasy") compared with the scan of a normal control subject; see p. 149 (McCann, Szabo, Scheffel, et al., 1988; reproduced courtesy of George Ricaurte, M.D.)

PLATE 17. "Plain Brain/Brain after Ecstasy"; an illustration for the Twenty-fifth Annivrsary Poster NIDA (National Institute of Drug Abuse); see p.150 (courtesy of NIDA)

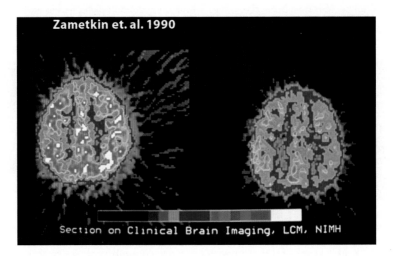

PLATE 18. PET scans of a patient with attention-deficit hyperactivity disorder (ADHD), compared with the scan of a normal control subject; see p.155 (courtesy of the National Institute of Mental Health)

. . . Then there was another kind of illness, as in, "God, she's a sick person," "How sick," "This is a really sick idea." The second kind carried the weight of moral blame. . . .

But what if depression was an illness of the first kind? Then it would be an incorrect functioning of my brain. I could say, *There is something wrong with my brain.* That was a different thing from saying, *There is something wrong with me.* The second was self-pitying; the first was a simple, factual statement. It was a subtle nuance, easy to miss. But as I grasped that difference — and it was slippery, I kept losing it at first — other doors began to open in my mind:

Depression is an illness. I am sick. I need to be here [in this mental institution] because I'm defective, not because I'm a moral leper, not because I've fallen from grace or turned my back on God, but for one simple reason: because I am sick.

But there my thinking stalled. So I was sick. But this was my *brain* I was talking about, not my gallbladder or my kidneys. It had some mysterious property called "consciousness." It produced behavior, the sum total of which was somehow *me.* If I wanted to say simply that my brain was sick, I could stop there and disavow responsibility for that sickness — but if I did that, I would be giving up my idea of autonomy in the world. I would be simply a product of some chemical abnormality in a lumpy gray organ between my ears. . . . It seemed to me that if the first approach was too simplistic, its opposite might be as well. (Thompson 1995, pp. 189–190)

Faced with the fact of her brain being sick, Thompson is *caught.* In some very real sense, she knows too much about her brain. Like Wittgenstein, she would be able to make sense of it if a connection were seen in her brain while reading. This also means, however, that if her brain is sick, she must be sick, too. How can she disavow her depression, then, without disavowing her self?

The solution Thompson eventually discovers is not to disavow either alternative but to create a new type of human, a depressed human, who is also a type of brain, a depressed brain. The invention in this case is carried out against her slippery notion of an ill person, but also morally sick, disgusting person. Out of this purely negative notion of sick (as not healthy and not good), she forges a positive identification with her own brain-illness. She *is* a depressed person because she *has* a depressed brain. The too-simple cultural alternatives of either being responsible for her sickness or not being her brain are complicated. She is her brain against her brain: She is now a person with depression fighting that depression. In her own metaphor, she is forever more wary of the Beast who travels with her. In this manner, given the stark choices of responsibility and autonomy, she enacts a powerful form of self-invention: identity politics. She comes to see herself as — and becomes — a particular kind of person, a kind she shares with others who also *have* depression and *are* people with depression. Beyond a shared affliction, all of these people share a brain-type that is a necessary response to social, historical, and institutional factors in the concerning the ongoing stigma attached to mental illness. Suffice it to note here the crucial enabling role played by both the NAMI in shaping research directions and public perceptions of mental illness as biological disease and of the Twelve-Step movement (an outgrowth of Alcoholics Anonymous) in establishing the positive identity of afflicted individuals as people who share a unique experience and are stronger for fighting it.[32]

Thompson's account illustrates three critical aspects of objective-self fashioning for our purposes. First, there is a tremendous flexibility and openness of explanation of the objective-self. Even in the face of specific received-facts about ourselves, there is room for negotiation and redefinition. Sociologists and anthropologists of psychology have called this the "pandemonium" of folk psychology. They also note, however, that even as we can play with mind and brain, motivation and behavior, we also ultimately must satisfy local common sense (Lutz 1988, p. 185).[33] For Thompson, the commonsense constraint consists in having to come up with a responsible relation *toward* her depression without being responsible *for* it. Attending to the active use of explanatory flexibility allows us to understand how "models serve social relations as much or more than social relations follow models" (Holland and Quinn 1987).

The second aspect of objective-self fashioning we need to highlight is the need for a nuanced, complex cultural, historical, and institutional — as well as scientific or biomedical — understanding of context. Objective-self fashioning is an ongoing process of social accounting to oneself and others in particular situations in which received-facts function as particularly powerful resources because they bear the objective authority of science. As the location of social accounting changes — to a lab, to a courtroom, to a doctor's office, to someone's home — the relative force of particular received-facts also changes.[34]

The third critical aspect of objective-self fashioning is the fundamental connection between the *brain* as objective-self and one's own personal identity. When genes are invoked as the cause of one's objective-self and aspects of one's personality, they can become a synecdoche for one's identity. If one has a gene for depression, one can fear *becoming* depressed. More troubling for Thompson, to the extent that it can be characterized and measured, the brain seems to *be* one's personal identity.[35] We can note here that brain images further confuse the part with the whole — even though brain images show only a slice of the brain, they show the slice as representing the whole brain, which in turn *is* the person. This contrast between genes and brains can be illustrated by reactions to images of the two. Emily Martin and Deborah Heath have noted that people with genetic afflictions hiss and boo at pictures of genes or enzymes thought to cause these afflictions (Heath 1997; Martin 1994, p. 16). Sufferers of mental illnesses do not react negatively to brain images of depression or schizophrenia. Rather, the reaction to brain images is often one of care and concern, much more akin to the reassurance and bonding experienced between parents and ultrasound images of fetuses. The brain image appears in this setting to be an image of the suffering of the afflicted, as well as an image of the affliction.[36]

The kind of brain that Thompson comes to understand is one that helps locate her Beast as a *brain-type*. Brain-types can stand for the human kind or state as their reality. Brain-types *fix*, and with imaging *show*, what is otherwise difficult to see, contested, or comes and goes.[37] Faced with a brain-type, a person is doubled as both being the brain-type and having it. Brain-types can conversely be said to *express* themselves in the person and as the person.

The relationship between Thompson and her brain appears to be a form of embodiment, but one not well studied in anthropology. Research on embodiment and the medicalized body have tended to oppose the two, with the lived, active body in opposition to the passive, objective, medical body (Becker 1995; Csordas 1994a; Csordas 1994b; Merleau-Ponty 1964). In the case of the brain in biomedical America, PET scan brain-types reveal a medicalized but active, unruly, and almost always irrational brain. Ironically, the "normal" brain-type is the one that is, so to speak, passive and lets the real self talk though it.[38] The depressed brain-type, however, substitutes itself for the real self and speaks instead, providing us with such an expression as "That was my illness speaking, not me," or in Thompson's terms, "That was the Beast." The brain-type, although objective, is simultaneously subjective, lived by the person as well as against the person.

Objective Self-Fashioning

> Given the explosive rate at which the fields of molecular genetics and neurobiology are expanding, it is inevitable that the perception of our own nature, in the field of sex as in all attributes of our physical and mental lives, will be increasingly dominated by concepts derived from the biological sciences.
> (LeVay 1993, pp. 137–138)

Within this broad sketch of three symbiotic actors—experts, laypersons, and mediators, each drawing on and reconfiguring the presuppositions of the others—I am going to concentrate my attention on the aspect I call objective self-fashioning. The objective self is an active category of the person that is developed through references to expert knowledge and invoked through facts. The objective self is also an embodied theory of human nature, both scientific and popular. Objective self-fashioning calls attention to the equivocal site of this production of new objective knowledge of the self. From one perspective, science produces facts that define who our selves objectively are, and which we then accept. From another perspective, our selves are fashioned by us out of the facts available to us through the media, and these categories of people are, in turn, the cultural basis from which new theories of human nature are constructed.

Objective self-fashioning is thus an acknowledgment of local mutations in categories of people highlighting the active and continual process of self-definition and self-participation in that process. Objective self-fashioning is how we take facts about ourselves — (about our bodies, minds, capacities, traits, states, limitations, propensities, and so on) — that we have read, heard, or otherwise encountered in the world and incorporate them into our lives.[39] As anthropologists and other scholars, we are most often in the mediator role, casting theories of objective selves out of our own categories of the person.

These cases point to two interrelated meanings of objective self-fashioning: (1) how we come to understand ourselves as subject to the scientific, medical, and technical discourses of objectivity, and (2) how these discourses choose "us" as their object of study. The difference between the two meanings is a matter of point of view. On the one hand, these cases point to the ways in which we fashion our selves — person, body, brain, and mind — out of ready-made objective types, and therefore subject ourselves to the disciplines of science and technology, expertise and machines. This kind of self encounters objectivity in the form of resistance; who we are is a product of discourse networks and technologies over which we have little control (Kittler 1985). On the other hand, the practices of science, technology, and medicine fashion selves as objective facts through scientific experimentation, subject selection, and medical taxonomic exercises. This latter case emphasizes social and disciplinary production of selves, whereas the former emphasizes cultural presuppositions built into concepts and practices.

Attending to the categories of the person built into facts, and to facts-in-the-world as facts, will enable us to see more clearly how medical and scientific claims, along with our own, are as much about dividing persons as they are about describing them. Here, along with Emily Martin, I believe we should also "acknowledge the varieties of ways in which experience resists science and medicine" (Martin 1987). More specifically, the question of objective self-fashioning raises the issue of creativity with regard to facts. Rayna Rapp, for instance, has followed the different ways in which people incorporate the possibilities and results of amniocentesis into their lives—for one mother, the fact of a genetic defect means a decision to abort, whereas for another, it means preparing to take proper care of a challenging baby (Rapp 1999). Both Martin and Rapp have called for a reader-response analysis of our relation to science, medicine, and other facts of life.

There are exceptions to this relief, of course. One senior PET researcher expressed his own fears regarding diagnosis by scan. Armed with detailed knowledge of how difficult it can be to produce an accurate image, he easily externalized the fact-producing technique from facts about himself:

> We've worked as hard as we can to make everything quantitative because almost everything you do to make it quantitative makes it a good picture, too. You don't have funny blobs. I don't know if you are familiar with some of the other kinds of imaging, but most of the images are just funny blobs that do not represent, in my mind, [the brain]. What you should see is a perfect image of the brain that has been blurred. If that is what you see, that means that you are doing it right. When you see funny blobs that are not part of it, you know they are screwing something up beyond having poor resolution.
>
> I find it difficult to have myself diagnosed by something like that. I'd be worrying that the blob on the right was a bad photomultiplier on the system and it wasn't really a problem. I guess there are some cases where the problem is so big and gross, a huge area missing, that you can do that. But I have to realize that everybody can't afford to do PET. It is scary that a lot of medicine, and a lot of tests, really are not all that great.

Within the daily practice of clinical psychiatry, these brain-imaging techniques have also helped sufferers deal with the fact of mental illness symptoms. The following excerpt is from an interview with Dr. Joseph Wu:

DUMIT: Do you show the patients their PET scans?

Wu: Oh yes. We try and show them the PET scans, and then some of these patients will refer them out to people. I have a part-time private practice with some of them, and they may like to continue with me.

DUMIT: Does it help them overcome part of the stigma of mental illness?

Wu: I think so. I think that [it] definitely [does]. One of the intrinsic messages is that the depression isn't something to be ashamed of; it

> is an illness which needs to be understood. And it is not something that is their fault.
>
> I think that there is a destigmatization that occurs with the biological emphasis. It is a fine line, because there are some arenas of personal responsibility that people can and should assume for their feelings. But I think it is a very narrow and tricky balance. It is important not to think that it is all biology; that it can lead to a certain eschewing of what is appropriate for one's own role in understanding one's emotions. On the other hand, I think that people can go overboard, and say, "Gee, I'm entirely at fault for how I feel." [It is important] to try and understand one's role in helping to monitor one's emotions without being unnecessarily harshly judgmental of oneself.

The reconfiguration of mental illness as biological through the use of PET scans becomes part of a personal reconfiguration of one's own category of person. A strict division between the biological self and the personal self is not at issue here. Rather, the relations between the two selves are redistributed so that although the patient must continue to experience the illness and live with it, she or he no longer has to identify with it. The diseased brain, in this case, becomes a part of a biological body that is experienced phenomenologically but is not the bearer of personhood. Rather, the patient who looks at his or her PET brain scan is an innocent sufferer rationally seeking help.[40]

Other researchers who have also shown patients their scans have agreed that especially in cases of neurological and mental diseases, which are often accompanied with self-disgust or a sense of failure, both the scan and the process help legitimate the problem. They make it something that can at least be explored.[41] These patients (and their families) want schizophrenia and depression to be medicalized, to have a single cause or explanation, even if there is no solution or cure for them.

Anthropologists of medicine have long explored this kind of effect as a crucial aspect of every health-care system. Jean Jackson discussed the failure of culture to come to grips with chronic pain (Good et al. 1992; Jackson 1994; Jackson 2000). The tension Jackson described involves the social devaluation of mental versus physical pain. Chronic pain sufferers seek out, even hope for, positive test results. They even hope for cancer, because then there would be something to point to and work on to solve the problem.

Regarding depression, Dr. Wu concurred with this interpretation when I asked him about the history of psychiatry.

> DUMIT: Dr. Wu, Nancy Andreasen has written about the biological revolution in psychiatry. You were in medical school during this time. Did you also get the other side of psychiatry?

WU: Oh, very much so. I would say that most of the psychiatrists in this department are still analytically, dynamically focused. I would say that biologically oriented psychiatrists still make up a minority of the faculty. Maybe thirty to forty percent, as opposed to the psychodynamically oriented people, [who] are fifty to sixty percent.

DUMIT: Do both of these sides come into play in your work?

WU: Somewhat. For me, when I do a study of depression, there is a part of me, a whole human dimension, that really tugs at my heart. Part of me feels moved by the pain of the patient that we work with. I am also moved by the courage and the willingness that many of these people have to participate in this study, even with the depth of their emotional pain and anguish. I think we try to offer to them the gratification that comes with knowing that they are contributing to the fund of knowledge that will eventually help to, we hope, eliminate depression or mitigate it. And that is something that many of these people find appealing, because there may be some greater purpose to their suffering. It is a way of reconnecting in some sense with the broader community. It is a way of making a personal meaning out of the emotional pain that they suffer from. For me, I see the whole biological aspect as not being contradictory or mutually exclusive from the psychodynamic aspect. I really see it as complementary and synergistic with the dynamic aspect. There are some people that see it as "either/ or." I see it more as a "both/and" type of proposition.

PET research into mental illness has thus become an area of study worthy of community support and patient contribution. The "both/ and" approach to psychiatry, popularized by books such as *Listening to Prozac*, involves realizing that the brain can be altered by the social environment and by genetic development and drugs. The kindling theory, for instance, suggests that repeated abuse during childhood can build up depressed reactions until the depression is neurologically self-sustaining.[42] The brain becomes "rewired" as if the person had been born that way. In the same vein, both psychodynamic talk therapy and psychopharmoceutical drug treatment can change brain chemistry and rewire the brain toward freedom from depression. Note that the brain remains the bearer of mental illness but in treatment becomes an intersection for social and biologic influences.

Dr. Wu's "both/and" approach to psychodynamic and biologic explanations of mental illness arises, I suspect, from his taking patients' perspectives into account. Patients can participate in social and medical reform by participating in research that might produce facts implying a category of person who suffers from a physiological rather than a psychologic disturbance.

If we see that responsibility and causations are part of our categories of people, this example demonstrates the flexibility and contestibility of these categories. Patients and activists are actively getting together to support and promote research on the shared biologic nature of mental illness because of their desire to see the results and their hope for cures. Paul Rabinow has called this grouping on the basis of biologic commonality "biosociality" (Rabinow 1992). A key point to remember here is that the facts of biology around which these groups are organizing are not necessarily fully decided within the scientific community. Yet they provide the means for social action, justifications for support of certain kinds of research, and arguments for a biologic understanding of mental illness. The facts enable the groups to further promote a category of the objective person that does not, in their view, prejudge them and condemn them to blame and guilt. This involves understanding the many very different ways facts (science, technology, nature) and experience (subjectivity, personality, culture) are constantly shaping and tripping over each other. These people are working creatively to refigure responsibility for mental illness, in this case to biology, in an attempt to gain control over this part of their world.

The challenge here is not just to the social construction of mental illness. This is not a simple story of the gradual emergence of the right view of depression, schizophrenia, and PET scanning. Biologic psychiatry, for instance, can lead to deinstitutionalization and differential access to medication, which burdens lower-income communities more than upper-income ones. This story is not one of victims and blame, however. By tracing facts-in-the-world throughout the virtual community of PET images, I hope that responsibility for these situations might be multiplied—that accountability might adhere to experts, mediators, and laypersons alike for their participation in objective self-fashioning.

Conclusion

When PET researcher Henry Wagner said that "in PET, we now have a new set of eyes that permits us to examine the chemistry of the human mind" (Wagner 1986, p. 253), he was pointing to a particular kind of humanoid: a cyborg whose experience of vision includes the physiology of the brain as witnessed through PET scanning. Some of us may shudder at the alienation implied in selves mediated by radiotracers, new pharmaceuticals, and multimillion-dollar bioscience. Others may breathe a sigh of relief at not being blamed for personally constructing schizophrenic children, at finally being respected as having wonderful children who happen to have a visible and therefore real brain dysfunction. Still others may wonder when and how they will be classed as normal or abnormal, or even if this binary categorization will finally prevail.

In conclusion, I have tried to point out some of the ways in which contemporary biomedical and scientific practices are culturally situated. These practices are participating in ongoing negotiations not just of specific brain–behavior–mind links but also of the nature of human nature and the significance of human differences. I have tried to show both the complexity of the process of producing contemporary neuroscientific facts and images and the numerous ways in which practical considerations often build in assumptions about human nature with undesirable and socially unequal consequences. My purpose is not to point a finger at any particular sets of people or techniques. I think it is necessary to recognize the social and cognitive benefits of these practices for many, many people. Rather, I am seeking to find a language to talk about multiple accountabilities between the diverse communities engaged with PET.

The challenges of how to understand the continuing and increasing presence of biotechnopower require close attention not only to the multiple uses and arenas of facts-in-the-world but also to their deployment within discourses of objectivity and to the ways that they have built-in, presupposed notions of human nature. The point is that science and medicine turn out to be our business on a daily basis. We are involved in them, they involve us, and they draw on the ways in which we configure the person. My hunch is that this process will reveal much about the multiple circuits of theory transfer from laypersons to experts and back again to laypersons via all kinds of mediators—movies, magazines, personal physicians, and anthropologists. These circuits of fact distribution and presupposition are worth understanding if we want to play a critical role in our own understanding of our selves.

WAGNER: You see, one of the appeals of activation studies is that it makes it possible to focus on particular parts of the brain for carrying out what I'm interested in, which is the neurochemistry, the molecular reactions that are going on. So therefore the activation studies are very interesting and very helpful. But from the example of circuit diagrams, of what is connected to what, what activates X is less interesting to me than the molecular approach.

DUMIT: How would you define the difference between these two kinds of studies?

WAGNER: Well, one is the area of molecular intercellular and intracellular communication. It's at the molecular level rather than at the regional level. So the activation lets you know that part of the temporal lobe is activated when you speak, and that another part of the brain is activated and associated with that. I think this is important and very interesting, and very useful in terms of focusing on what is going on.

But then you want to see exactly *how* information is stored in your brain (figure 5.2). I think people are—I know I certainly am—more conscious of the effects of molecules on your brain than we ever have been before. People's way of thinking becomes automatic. I think people realize that chemicals are affecting your brain all of the time. I'm conscious of the fact that if you feel a certain way at a certain time, [then] if you wait a little while, these chemicals are going to be making adjustments, just as neurotransmitters are going to be leaving receptors and they will be available for more stimulation. You see, I am much more conscious now of chemistry going on in my brain, and everybody else's brain, than I was when we started doing this.

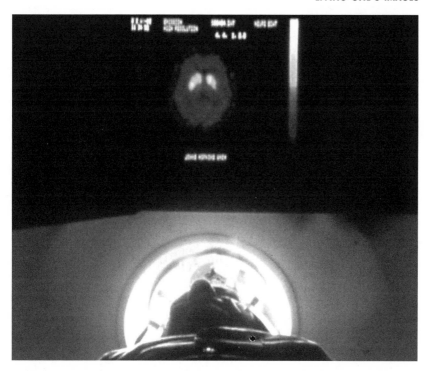

FIGURE 5.2. Henry N. Wagner, M.D., shown in PET scanner. His brain image (above) shows dopamine receptor density. (Original slide provided by Dr. Wagner)

Chapter 6

Conclusion: Here Is a PET Image of a Person That Shows Depression

This book could have begun with the following declaration: Here is a PET image of a person that shows depression. The book could have taken off from there and described the consequences for theories of depression and human nature on the basis of scan results. As an anthropologist of science and technology, however, I was compelled to write a book that first took apart, unpacked, and analyzed each aspect of the declaration and its relation to the world.

The reference of "PET" had to be examined historically, in terms of what PET is and does (chapter 2). Before a PET image could be "here," it had to come from somewhere else, from an experiment, and for it to be an "image of" something, a visual semiotics had to be explored (chapter 3). For a PET image to "show" a truth about a person, a interrogation of the social contract of technological human measurement had to be set forth (chapter 4). For there to be an image "of a person," the nature of personhood had, at least, to be interrogated in relation to knowledge production and dissemination. Finally, for a mental illness like depression to be the object of such a technological measurement, the social actors and consequences involved in such a process had to be explored (chapter 5). None of these projects is completed, but each has been started in such a way that cultural connections among the long list of actors in the virtual community of PET images may be accounted for. A rich history of the contests over PET and its objects can now be begun and a rich inquiry into a particular set of experiments can be initiated.

As anthropologists and historians relatively informed about the virtual community of PET, we could now track how in these experiments the PET scanner was justified, the experiment was designed, the patients and normal control subjects were selected, the data were generated, the images were selected and then argued for, and what hypotheses were generated or confirmed about the nature of depression and human nature. In doing this, however, we must go further than noting the assumptions about human nature, the brain, and mental illness being invoked. Each of these assumptions has its own histories and contests that are difficult to bring into focus so long as the content of PET remains opaque. How to juggle approaches to brain imaging and philosophies of human nature remains a most elusive and yet crucial problem for the neurosciences.

For the rest of this conclusion, I would like to explore the nature of such an inquiry, beginning with the statement "Here is a PET image of a person that shows depression." The following comments from a discussion with neurologist and medical imaging researcher Helen Mayberg offer a starting point.

> I have always been surprised that there haven't been more studies on depression, because it is such a common problem. Even though I myself do not suffer from depression, I feel a real empathy and curiosity about depression and mood. Everybody has moods. And they can be so incapacitating. Everybody experiences grief, everybody has disappointments in life. What are these? Even when you know what is going on, you can't shake it. What is that?
>
> But then to actually look at sadness — depressed people are sad, normal people are sad — how do these things interact? What is the circuitry that regulates just the experience of sadness? This circuitry is interesting both as a confound to the disease and as part of a bigger picture. We are trying to hammer out what the distributed network that regulates mood looks like, whether it be a normal or [an] abnormal mood.

For Mayberg, depression is both a disease (not part of normal life) and an emotion (sadness, part of normal life), so her experiments have to be designed to discover the appropriate components of each: How might normal emotion mask a disease, and how is the disease itself a kind of abnormal emotion? In other words, is sadness continuous or discontinuous with depression? Is depression, for example, being normally sad but for too long, or too deeply or inappropriately? Or is it a different kind of sadness from normal sadness? Might there even be depression without sadness?[1] These questions, she pointed out, require the biological and cultural nature of emotions — in this case, the circuitry or distributed network regulating moods — to be delineated (figure 6.1).

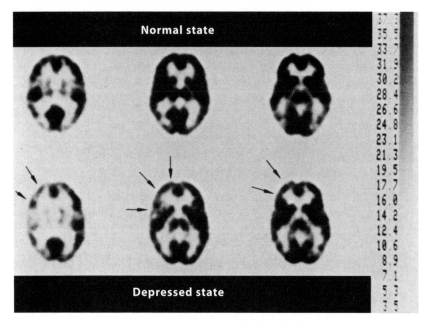

FIGURE 6.1. Normal and depressed states. Original caption reads: "Images obtained with the NeuroECAT tomograph using the fluorodeoxyglucose (FDG) method to measure local cerebral glucose metabolism. The gray scale is proportional to the glucose metabolic rate with the black being the highest. The top row of images is from an age-matched control subject. The bottom row of images is from a patient with unipolar depression. In the patient study, note the left-to-right metabolic asymmetry of the perisylvian frontotemporal cortex, which extends to the superior temporal zone. This pattern of glucose metabolism has been seen in some but not all patients with unipolar depression." (From Phelps et al. 1975, reproduced with permission)

Already histories and cultural categories of mood and emotions, and sadness and depression must be investigated.[2] Are emotions being opposed to rationality and practical reasoning[3] or are they included as aspects of all activity, providing reason and action their colors? Norbert Wiener, for instance, suggested that "the stored information of the mind lies on many levels of accessibility and is much richer and more varied than that which is accessible by direct unaided introspection; that it is vitally conditioned by affective experience" (Wiener 1961, p. 149 quoted in Heims 1991, p. 150). Cross-cultural studies of both emotions and emotional and mental abnormalities must also be consulted.[4] Regional and national differences also cannot be ignored.[5]

If mood is to be delineated in itself (as a distributed network), what moods are to be included? Greimas and Fontanille's *Semiotics of Passions* might provide a useful grid or taxonomy for unpacking pathemic components specific to U.S. sadness. They explicitly raised the real problem of the epistemology of passions, distinguishing modalities of mood — sentiment, emotion, humor, likeliness, inclination, temperament, and character — via different combinations of disposition (permanent, durable, temporary), manifestation (continuous, episodic, isolated), modalization (knowing, being-able, wanting, mixed), and competence (acknowledged, supposed, negated).[6] They explicitly note that "[n]omenclature is, in a sense, a first draft, an intuitive product of history, of a theory of passions developed within a culture" (Greimas and Fontanille 1993, p. 52).[7] Consulting Irigaray and Descartes, we might ask whether "wonder" is to be considered the first passion or, instead, the key to rationality led by curiosity[8] (What of the feeling of the sublime?) Key to this kind of analysis would be understanding the possibilities and problems various types of tasks evoke in culturally embodied persons. Parts of this line of questioning are pursued by Mayberg:

MAYBERG: An important experiment is to examine what happens in the brain when normal people are sad, whether their brains change in the same ways that brains of depressed people do. There have been several reports on this. José Pardo, when he was at Washington University, found certain areas of the brain had increased blood flow in normal people thinking sad thoughts. And Mark George, at [the National Institute of Mental Health], reported something very similar in normal people thinking sad thoughts while looking at sad faces.

We used a different tactic. We felt that to see brain changes specific for mood, you had to separate out the cognitive component from the experiential component. As you design a PET scanning experiment, you are trying to compartmentalize behavior into its component parts as best you can [on the basis of] the scientific data that is available. If you can, you always try to have a stepwise progression of complexity. Or the alternative is that you take complex behavior and you try to break it down into its individual behavioral parts. So how do you know when you have the most basic pieces?

DUMIT: No factors left.

MAYBERG: Exactly. My collaborator, Mario Liotti, M.D., Ph.D., and I decided, "Look, we don't want a scan of just *thinking* sad thoughts — we want a scan of *sadness*." So our design was to avoid doing a scan while they were thinking; we wanted to get them into the "altered state," if you will, and then do the scan. And we got the opposite of what has been reported [by both Pardo and George]. Our "normal people being sad" looked like "depressed people." The flow goes down in the same regions, and it is very selective. There are also some areas that go up, the most interesting being in the anterior cingulate. Those areas are the focus of our present work.

Two paradigms of sadness are presented here: thinking sad thoughts and being sad. In the experiments done at Washington University, for instance, subjects were asked to *think* deeply about sad events and rated themselves on how sad they became. Holding off for a moment who is selected and what is meant by "sad," already an extreme difference has been located. Scanning normal people who "are sad" and therefore in an "altered state" of mind produces a kind of opposite effect from normal people who think sad thoughts. Each is distinct, and each is different. In one of the "thinking sad thoughts" experiments, some researchers considered the possibility of taking sad thinking to its limits. They thought of getting method actors, who theoretically can think themselves into being sad.[9] Each of these experiments now becomes a different piece in a growing puzzle.

Each of these experiments, by studying all of these different things related to mood, you start to . . . it's like you have these transparencies that overlap in some areas but not others, and you keep laying down these layers, one experiment after the other. All of a sudden, you start to get some overlap and you also start to see some things in some areas that you hadn't even suspected. That has led us to building a model of a distributed network regulating mood that can explain the sort of co-morbid presentation of mood and attentional deficits in depressed people, and how to potentially compartmentalize these clinical features. Because depression has cognitive elements. What does that mean? Obviously normal sadness taps into memory, taps into attention, taps into a lot of things. It is no big surprise that when you whack out part of that system, with whatever causes depression, that you are going to have an impact on much more than just being sad. And what is that? How is sadness different in depressed people and nondepressed people? This is where we are now in terms of the work.

As Mayberg and her colleagues' models of sadness and depression develop through these experiments, they branch out "visually" (via the images of brain locations activated by sadness), into "attention," "memory," and so on. By being careful, Mayberg is also required to become a full-fledged philosopher, developing her own philosophical (or physiological) anthropology.[10] This of course, has been an underlying theme of this entire book: To perform a PET experiment is already to be engaged in a philosophical anthropology.

Projects that study human functions or powers or faculties are as old as medicine.[11] As mentioned earlier, PET researchers have often pointed to phrenology as a key historical period when the right questions were being asked with the wrong technology. For these contemporary function mappers, or network trackers, then, the functions that they decide are possible to delimit will determine the nature of human nature that they discover. Steven Kosslyn, for example, in his book *Wet Mind: The New Cognitive Neuroscience*, attended to them in the following manner. Out of 422 pages of his text, he devoted 91 percent to traditional cognitive neuroscience:

Table 6.1a
Wet Mind

Chapter Titles	Number of Pages	Percent of Pages
Computation	35	8
Visual Perception	76	18
Visual Cognition	39	9
Reading	44	10
Language	75	18
Movement	55	13
Memory	60	14

In his final chapter, "Gray Matters," Kosslyn explored what he left out earlier:

Table 6.1b
Wet Mind, *Continued*

Subsection Titles	Number of Pages	Percent of Pages
Reasoning	7	2
Arithmetic	5	1
Cerebral Lateralization	13	3
Consciousness	7	2
Emotion	2	0.5
Rehabilitation	4	1

Kosslyn's emphasis was clearly on what we might call clear cognitive processing, as opposed to unclear—gray—social matters. The section on consciousness is devoted to whether consciousness exists or not, and how it might exist. Presumably (though he did not talk about them), curiosity, sexuality, violence, caring, friendship, religiosity, play, and so on fit somewhere under "emotion." I asked Mayberg about my perception of these kinds of projects:

DUMIT: I was just reading Kosslyn's book, *Wet Mind*, looking at these cognitive neuroscientists who play with PET. In this book he has 420 pages on the brain and two pages on emotions, forty pages on visual cognition, seventy-five on perception. The more I looked around, the more it struck me [that for] these cognitive neuroscientists, [so much of] their view of what the person *is* comes down to these microprogram notions of cognition. I guess what I was wondering whether this difference is due to who had access to PET first.

MAYBERG: No, I don't think it is. I think that in classical thinking, theories about emotions are very noncompartmentalized.[12] The idea of a brain localization for emotions is very unsettling to many people. I used to get into fights when I would talk about what I wanted to study, because people don't necessarily like the idea that something like emotion can be compartmentalized to some spot or group of spots in the brain. Just the idea that very, very personal behaviors have some kind of neuron-to-neuron analog is somehow disconcerting.

More of an issue though, I think, is that in terms of classical, cognitive neuroscience, you deal with things that can be broken down into component parts. Successful cognitive neuroscience is able to do that.

Emotions experiments are just harder to put into the cognitive neuroscience model. Emotions don't easily fit into these constructs. They are confounded by memory, attention, motion behaviors, and so on. So it becomes: "I don't think I can design a good experiment, and I don't want to be a loser, and I don't want to produce meaningless or uninterpretable results."

Many of the people who do study emotion look at descriptive phenomenology, even if they have very well-constructed paradigms. Unfortunately, there is not a lot to hang your hat on. With vision experiments, it is very different. We know about shapes; we know about color; we know about movement. The researcher can say, "Okay, now we have to look in the various visual fields; now we have to look at directed attention; now we have to look . . ." One can start to add together these individual components. With emotion, it is hard to get a handle on where to start. What has happened is that we've pretty much jumped in feet first and are starting to sort out the details.

There certainly are a lot of people who study emotion. But in terms of having paradigms that can be easily and successfully translated into an imaging experiment, I think it is harder to do than for some of these other behaviors like vision, motion, and language.

Artificial emotions?[13] Mayberg raises two fascinating cultural issues about personhood. One is that we [who?] do not easily think of emotions (in particular) or emotion (in general) along the same lines of compartments or programs, that we do with rational action and sensation. We can imagine intelligence working like a computer, but we cannot imagine a program for sadness. In fact, the computer is often pointed to precisely as the embodiment of emotionlessness! Likewise, the sensorium is based on a model of information-processing and is conceivable as a set of programs for analyzing and distinguishing objects,[14] though, of course, we have to work hard to make pain fit this metaphor.[15]

Regarding emotions, one must eventually make some sort of human function argument, often dependent on an argument from an evolutionary purpose (or evolutionary side effect). Why did humans evolve with emotions? It is here where various anthropologies (biological, archaeological, physical, cultural, medical) are often employed as facts to explain the data.[16]

Mayberg's other observation about the difficulty of locating and studying emotions in the brain is located specifically and historically within cognitive psychology. As historians of statistics have shown, the functions emphasized have been those easy to isolate and repeat—those, in other words, that could be made to produce bell curves.[17]

What is the connection, we might ask, between these two difficulties? How are the simple-mechanism studies emphasized and popularized by cognitive psychology related to thinking about the brain as an emotionless computer? One aspect of computer networks, for instance, is that the faster they work, the better. Theoretically, they take no time: In an ideal neural-network model of vision, for instance, a bunch of colored dots and contrast gradients are recognized (immediately) as a picture of a horse. Emotions, however, make sense only within time. Heidegger described moods as that state which one is always already "thrown into."[18] In this sense, emotions are more easily conceived of by the analogy to a disease—a change in the state of a person—than by the analogy to a computer network. This distinction between being sad and thinking sad thoughts, however, is one already made by Mayberg et al.

Still, the metaphor of a network that processes or transmits information remains confusing. PET scans, as currently conceived, inherently seem to show only activity on a one-dimensional scale: either more or less activity than normal.

DUMIT: It is interesting how when these results go from the experiment and the scientific article, where everything is very careful, to the popular media, the question of what is being studied gets transformed. It seems to me quite difficult to convey what is being depicted in these images.

POSTDOCTORAL PET RESEARCHER: Yes! The things that we are measuring, it is not necessarily that glucose utilization is directly related at all to oxygen consumption, nor that these two parameters are directly related to electrical activity. And even if they were related, it is not necessarily true that electrical activity is related to the amount of information that is transmitted by neurons. It is not. If a neuron is firing more, it does not mean that it is transmitting more information, because in epilepsy, for example, the neurons are firing a huge amount. It is meaningless to think of firing in terms of information. If you are looking for neurons in terms of information, you have what are called "spiking neurons." You have regular striking and you have bursts. Spiking neurons are those that if you give them a stimulus, a square pulse, of a certain length, they will give a single action potential. Regular striking [ones], you give them the same pulse, you get four or five action potentials. They will appear at a frequency of twenty to thirty Hertz. With bursting neurons, they will give you a burst of action potentials, which will ride on a kind of depolarizing wave. So if now we are trying to ask, "Where do I have more information?" the common idea is that with bursting neurons you have less information transmitted than with spiking ones. But again, it is a kind of question which is just a hypothesis. We are just able to measure action potentials. To try to convert it, or compare it to signals that are coming through a telephone cable . . . maybe it is true! No doubt it is quite effective, because this guy is living in a world with telephone cables [referring to Roger Sherrington's famous metaphor of the brain like a telegraph]. It doesn't mean that there is something we know about the brain. The brain was created some millions of years before telephone cables were created. Who knows, maybe we created telephone cables just because in our mind, maybe our brain works like this! All of these things are just hypotheses. I wouldn't even jump to the conclusion. First of all I would try to define what learning [is]. Then beyond that, do exercises affect development of the brain? I think that is a good question. But to go beyond this kind of thing . . . I think that in the future we will have a lot of studies, very clever kinds of studies, that will try to give us better answers about intelligence and that sort of thing.

In a fascinating and dizzying trail of thoughts, this researcher works backward from PET scan to neuronal activity to some of the original studies for defining and measuring this activity (evoked potentials). The metaphor on which all of these technologies depend — an equation of quantity of information with size of the potential — he notes, is based on a historically situated technology: electrical information in telephone wires.[19] Which came first, he wonders, the metaphor of neuronal activity or the neuronal activity of the metaphor? The solution, he concludes, is not to look for a conclusion now, but to further break down the problem, get to work, and to look forward to the future.

Many layers of metaphors are embedded in notions of information as quantifiable, as something that is communicated via a code that can be cracked, and as the substrate of language and social information that is processed. Unpacking the implications of these notions that underlay theories of the brain should be a central part of the kind of project proposed in this chapter.

With emotions, of course, neurotransmitters play a bigger role than with traditional cognitive psychology.[20] Each neurotransmitter has its traditional faculty. Henry Wagner spoke to me about some of the pros and cons of this legacy with regard to using neurotransmitter experiments to think about diseases:

> To divide the brain function up into cognition and emotion and movement is again an example of categorization that is probably not too helpful with depressed patients. Alzheimer's patients can be depressed, and depressed patients have trouble thinking, and schizophrenic patients can have trouble moving — they can become catatonic. These are very broad categories. And I personally believe that putting anything into a category should be done not because there is some kind of intrinsic truth to it but because it is useful. My philosophy is pragmatic. And therefore when you say that a person has disease X, it should be because putting him in that pigeonhole makes a difference in some way. These are man-made categories: abstractions are man-made simplifications of an unbelievably complex external world. Therefore, to say that dopamine has to do with movement — it has a lot to do with movement, but it has a lot to do with other things as well.
>
> What science does is try to make everything more and more simple, [to] try and get more common factors to get it simpler. But right now, in the area of mental function and mental disease, it is not very simple. So the goal is to try and come up with some kind of simple explanation for these things. Right now, you say you have a simple explanation where serotonin is related to mood and dopamine is related to movement and acetylcholine is related to learning or intelligence. But to say that acetylcholine is intelligence, serotonin is mood,

and dopamine is movement is a gross and unhelpful simplification, a counterproductive simplification. Although it is true that blocking the dopaminergic system has been one way that it has been found to help some patients with schizophrenia, and blocking the serotonin uptake site or inhibiting monoamine oxidase has been one way of helping patients become less depressed. If it helps, it helps. It helps solve problems. The world is surrounded with problems; people are surrounded with problems. *If an abstraction helps them — the best invention of all is language. I think that the most important part of consciousness and memory is language, because it translates the past into the present.*

Once again, philosophical anthropology must be brought explicitly into the discussion in order to proceed. We could here set Henri Bergson's (1988) reflections on physiology, memory, and language side by side with Wagner's and read both through Friedrich Kittler's (1985) analysis of turn-of-the-nineteenth-century attempts to map the languages of the subconscious using traditional cognitive psychology or through contemporary PET experiments mapping "language" (usually Indo-European) and "memory."[21]

Finally, let us look at one more aspect of Mayberg's description, the idea that she is looking into "the distributed network that regulates mood." The ease with which either a network or mood can be spoken of within neuroscience as *regulated* belies a long history within and without physiology on this concept. Canguilhem, the historian and philosopher of science, has followed this conceptual history of "regulation" and how it entered physiology. For medicine in particular, it made sense, because "people became ill and recovered all the time . . . [providing] a sense that the body hid inherent restitutive powers" (Canguilhem 1988). This notion of a dynamic, self-regulating system, Canguilhem noted, predates the autoimmune system and should also be seen as ontologically at odds with notions of coding errors. Coding-error models presume that an error leads to poor regulation. Recovery from error becomes the problem. On the self-regulatory model, however, recovery from error is the presumption.[22]

One researcher I talked to who studies neurotransmitters described the brain as having two million functions. "If any one is up or down, then it is dysfunctional." However, he said, the most important thing to study is the adaptive functions of the brain. When one neurotransmitter agonist is introduced, another system immediately kicks in, and another. The only way to study the brain is to try to capture each of these microreactions. "It makes for very frustrating nights," he confessed, "but it is also much more exciting." Regarding depression, he elaborated a specifically autoregulatory model in which the environment was an important component. "For everyone with depression, there are many, many more with the same kinds of brain but who have adapted." He suggested that depression is perhaps a failure of or loss of the ability to adapt. Depression as a state, then, is something that we might be continually cycling in and out of rapidly, our brains adapting with myriad systems of self-regulation. Becoming depressed, however, means not that something special has happened, or there has been a breakdown, but rather there is no longer the ability to so adapt quickly to these same conditions that before were "normal" ebbs and flows.

Other researchers who also subscribe to molecular and neurochemical views of the brain use the more current metaphor[23] of a coding error:

DUMIT: In some sense, with this new department, from this interdisciplinary program, you are trying to cement a new kind of discipline together.

PHELPS: That is right. It is called the Department of Molecular and Medical Pharmacology. This is a very natural thing, you know, when you think about it. Pharmacology as a discipline began to fail in many ways as a discipline. If you go back about three decades ago, [when] pharmacology began, the major activity in pharmacology was neuropharmacology. It was a time of grind and bind, doing assays of neurotransmitter systems. That is how neuropharmacology became very popular and very productive. It was teaching a lot of new things about the brain, and drug companies had focused on the brain and were developing drugs for the brain. And pharmacology became the acting accountant for that. But then neuroscience was born, and neuroscience in a decade went from a group of maybe twenty-five, thirty people to fourteen thousand. And to form neuroscience, it went into physiology and said, "Give me your neuroscientists." It went into anatomy and pharmacology and collected out the neuroscience people. Well, in pharmacology, that was particularly devastating, because the best and the majority of people were neuroscientists. So they left, they went out. And pharmacology started to lose its way. And that was kind of ironic, because out in the real world the drug industry had recognized a great opportunity in modern biology and biotechnology for the development of new drugs. And in fact, a lot of academic people recognized the opportunity to deliver something important to the public and also make a lot money doing it. So they took ideas and formed startup companies — Genentech, Amgen — and now many companies have driven biology and biotechnology to develop new

183

drugs. Well, that had a very fundamental basis, actually, because out of all this biology, they were shifting emphasis onto basic mechanisms by which the genome produces proteins, produces those proteins organized into a biochemical system to run itself. But while they were doing it, people were coming in, finding the errors of disease, fundamental errors. So then the concept started to develop to understand the molecular regulation of the cell, identify the molecular errors of disease and develop molecular corrections. That is, if there is an error in the genetic code, knock it out. If there is an error in a message that is being transcribed by the messenger RNA, then develop a drug to block that message. So now a whole new class of drugs were being developed that would focus on a whole new set of protein targets, and now a generation would be born that would master molecular corrections of disease. Well, they're drugs. The industry was moving a lot faster than pharmacology was. It was lagging behind.

But it is more than that. Everything originates and is carried out through chemistry and biology. What you think is structure is really that portion of biology that says we have to build and maintain a framework, and within this framework we will go and do things. If you look at disease, all disease starts by an error in the chemical process. All disease. And it typically goes about eroding away the reserves, and compensatory capability of that biological system to accommodate that normal process. But eventually, if the person becomes symptomatic, it has eroded away the reserves; there is no further way to compensate. So now the cellular function begins to fail. But like any system, it is designed to accommodate a lot of changes.

These two metaphors of autoregulation and coding are not necessarily opposed, as Phelps suggested at the end, but each implies different consequent interpretations of data results, and even of automatic programmed data analysis. For instance, the former involves multiple neurotransmitter regulations, actions, and reactions, whereas the latter is more amenable to a brain-mapping, interrupted-circuit interpretation. One of the questions that must be addressed is the continued coexistence of these different metaphorics. This is no simple or even complicated historical change. The answer, I suggest, lies in the analysis of specific problems with specific technologies (and at specific institutions). Each brings with and builds into the results layers of tropes and kinds of personhood.

A further issue, related to all of these metaphors of interrelated circuits or systems, is how to justify stopping the set of significant communicating systems at the skin. The environment and sociality have to be seen as also in communication with these systems "in the brain." Rhythms, especially diurnal and seasonal patterns related to light, are just one place to examine such interaction. The field of psychoneuroimmunology has proposed an entire paradigm of illness based on elaborate socio-environmental circuits of communication (Levin and Solomon 1990).

Understanding a PET image of a person with depression requires, then, reflection on categories of people and metaphors of the brain, as well as imaging technologies and practices. Suffice it to acknowledge here the tremendously rich and potent work being done with PET scanning: careful and speculative, exciting and troubling. I hope I have made it clear in this book that much reflective work remains to be done as PET grows clinically, popularly, scientifically, and forensically. There are obligations and accountabilities regarding imaging practices as much as there are regarding selection procedures and consent forms.

At the 1991 meeting of the Society for Neuroscience, a plenary talk was given by Louis Sokoloff, one of the fathers of nuclear medicine. He began his talk with a wry acknowledgment and admonishment regarding the power of functional images: "We know we need to hype to get our grants. Let's try to keep it out of our results!" The "hype" surrounding these images must be understood as consonant with the fact that PET functional brain imaging is still a basic research project (as opposed to an applied one), and therefore survives on its ability to market its potential to particular audiences.[24] The meaning and presentation of these images are not at all decided among the imaging "experts"; and their debates deal directly with the issues I have been raising, if not always in the same terms. Questions about the significance of human brain variability — and whether to present typical images or average images or subtraction images — are thoroughly about mind–brain philosophies and the significance of human kinds. In functional brain imaging, the concepts of brain causation, human distinction, and mind functions are in flux and being actively renegotiated out of past and popular conceptions.

I would like to claim, or propose, that with brain function imaging, we, in the United States, may have entered a space of active negotiation of the basic terms of our categories of the person. This is a negotiation already underway with respect to ultrasound, the human genome project, HIV testing status, amniocentesis, and so on, but with a new emphasis on didactic images.[25] The court battles over the admissibility of these images are just beginning. The use of these images in thinking about ourselves is in its infancy. *We* are at stake in this work. How can we not afford to risk jumping in and studying it?

185

Notes

Chapter 1

1. The best source for clinical PET information is the Academy of Molecular Imaging (http://www.ami-imaging.org), especially the Institute for Clinical PET within it.

2. The recent book *Clinical Positron Emission Tomography (PET): Correlation with Morphological Cross-Sectional Imaging* bears out this observation. In addition to chapters on coronary artery disease and various cancers, it contains only three chapters on clinical PET imaging of the brain: brain tumors, epilepsy, and dementias (Schulthess 2000).

3. The new history of the brain is just beginning. Classics include Harrington (1987) and Star (1989) on localization; Jeannerod (1985); Smith (1992); and Deleuze (1989) on philosophy.

4. Unlike explicit ideologies of blame, hegemonic ones are difficult to trace to human agents. This notion of ideology is similar to Althusser (1984, 1976), especially as extended by Pêcheux (1982).

5. We keep a hyphen in *objective-self* because we need to highlight the fact that it refers to how we are to ourselves and to society an object of science and medicine, not how we "objectively" are to science and medicine. Our concern thus centers around the *object* of science and medicine, not their *methods* — not what justifies mental illness, but how it is specified by a set of practices, documents, institutions that enable it to be "objective." On the study of the object of science and medicine in this manner, see Rajchman (1985).

6. The caption for the images reads: "Looking at 'slices' of the brain in action: pictures made by the latest radiology miracle-machine PETT VI (Positron Emission Transaxial Tomograph), *right*. These brain scans show — graphically — how a normal brain's function compares with that of a depressed or schizo-

phrenic patient's; red line in the drawing *above* indicates CM + 5 plane depicted in the three scans. Slides from Brookhaven National Laboratory and New York University Medical Center."

7. STS (science and technology studies) work on these areas includes (Biagioli et al. (1994), Bourdieu (1975), Latour (1987).

8. Scientists work in a nonpassive world; see (Downey and Dumit (1997a), Hess (1995), and Martin (1994). On the activity of the social world, Franklin and Ragone (1998) wrote that "representations are themselves technologies of reproducing and transforming worlds."

9. On the historical development of our modern notions of the fact, see Poovey (1998), Porter (1995), and Shapin and Schaffer (1985). Whitehead (1938) provides a critical view of how we live with facts that nevertheless acknowledges precisely this notion of objective fashioning: "A single fact in isolation is the primary myth required for finite thought. This mythological character arises because there is no such fact. It follows that in every consideration of a single fact there is the suppressed presupposition of the environmental coordination requisite for its existence."

10. Such studies are conducted by physicists (Galison 1997; Gusterson 1996; Knorr-Cetina 1999; Traweek 1988) and microbiologists (Fleck 1979; Keller 1983; Latour 1987; Latour and Woolgar 1979). For overviews of the many debates over the production of facts in STS, see Ashmore (1989), and Lynch (1993).

11. Portions of my interviews are collected in Dumit (1995b). Labs visited include Washington University in St. Louis, Johns Hopkins University, Brookhaven National Laboratory, Massachusetts General Hospital, University of California, Los Angeles, and the University of California, Irvine. Conferences included those of the Radiological Society of North America, Society for Neuroscience, Society of Nuclear Medicine, and Organization for Human Brain Mapping.

12. "A central organizing question in ethnography should be to interpret what is at stake for particular persons in particular situations" (Kleinman and Kleinman 1991). See also Bourdieu (1990).

13. This book represents the anthropological work I have done. My historical work is discussed in chapter 2 ("Metaphors, Histories, and Visions of PET"). The full history of PET remains to be written.

14. A major problem in judging or even reporting these accusations was elegantly summed up by Jean-Pierre Changeux (who was reflecting on debates over phrenology) in *The Neuronal Man*: "As is often the case, an ideological debate grew into a controversy based on deficient technique" (Changeux 1985).

15. See Fischer (1995) and the *Late Editions* series of books edited by George Marcus for further discussions of the use of excerpted interview materials, especially Marcus (1995).

16. On evocation in ethnography, see Tyler (1987). Tyler's descriptions are the starting point for Strathern (1991).

17. See especially *On Certainty* (OC), *Last Writings on Psychology*, *Zettel*, and *Philosophical Investigations*. (PI). "As children we learn facts; e.g., that every human being has a brain, and we take them on trust." (OC, p. 159). " 'I

know that I am a human being.' In order to see how unclear the sense of his proposition is, consider its negation. At most it might be taken to mean 'I know I have the organs of a human.' (E.g., a brain which, after all, no one has ever yet seen.) But what about such a proposition as 'I know I have a brain.'? Can I doubt it? Grounds for doubt are lacking! Everything speaks in its favour, nothing against it. Nevertheless it is imaginable that my skull should turn out empty when it was operated on." (*OC*, p. 4).

18. *OC*, §204. Wittgenstein spends much time trying to specify the nature of our practice of coming to an end, somewhere between grounds and logic. Explanations come to an end (*PI*, I, p. 87). "Doesn't testing come to an end?" (*OC*, p. 164). For another take on this process, see Dumit (2000b).

Chapter 2

1. Another researcher, cited in chapter 3, directly compares PET scanning to participant observation.

2. In one of the inaugural introductions of PET to the broader research community in the journal *Science*, Phelps and Mazziotta note that though "there are limitations . . . and we must recognize that ambiguity can arise . . . the ability to make such measurements in the living human brain more than compensates for the extensive developmental work which is required in the validation of a new PET method." (Phelps and Mazziotta 1985, p. 802)

3. Similarly structured articles include Maisey (1989), and Nice (1980).

4. For a detailed review of phrenology, see Clarke and Jacyna (1987), pages 212–307. A partial list of some phrenological areas include:

> amativeness, philoprogenitiveness, concentrativeness, adhesiveness, combativeness, destructiveness, secretiveness, acquisitiveness, constructiveness, self-esteem, love of approbation, cautiousness, benevolence, veneration, conscientiousness, firmness, hope, wonder, ideality, wit, imitativeness, individuality, form perception, size perception, weight perception, colour perception, locality perception, number perception, order perception, memory of things, time perception, tune perception, linguistic perception, comparative understanding, and metaphysical spirit. (*Encyclopedia Brittanica*, "Phrenology," 1995)

5. Harrington is responding to a question regarding the dominant foothold of Norman Geshwind's 1960s localization model of connecting pathways whose interruption results in this or that syndrome.

6. With the brain, the competition between notions of data is particularly acute. Roberts (1991) reported that the Human Brain Project's attempt to think through a database for the brain "will be incredibly difficult. . . . Genome project informatics is trivial by comparison." This comment is by Peter Pearson, who directs the Genome Data Base at Johns Hopkins University. The following is a comment by one researcher I interviewed, concerning his experiences as a database designer trying to find a conceptual meeting place for different kinds of neuroscientists:

Even with fifty million dollars, you couldn't do all things that were needed by everybody, you couldn't satisfy the needs of the neuroscientists who wanted to look at micron-sized objects, and at the same time satisfy the objectives of people who wanted to look at the brain as a whole and map the functions and the anatomy. . . . So I think that there was that tension. There was also tension with the people who were interested in the behavior of individual neurons and how a synapse works. Therefore, if they do a brain map, they want something at a micron and submicron resolution.

7. Comparability is also the subject of much debate. For instance, see Poeppel (1996) and the discussion in this text that follows over the question of what constitutes overlapping results in the brain. Beaulieu (2000) discusses the attempts to create collective atlas-based databases of results.

8. See Andreasen (1989), Kereiakes (1987), Phelps (1991), Reivich and Alavi (1985), and Ter-Pogossian (1992).

9. Gewertz is quoted in Krech (1991). Krech reviews the contested history of ethnohistory, revealing a host of different meanings and approaches. I cling most strongly to the cultural anthropological definition outlined in the following quote: "To decipher history, one must appreciate the different ways people 'imagine the past'; one must be attentive to narratives . . . one must understand how history 'is both a metaphor of the past and a metonymy of the present' (75:2); and one must be aware of the perspective-dependent and contested nature of histories (159, 241) or of the variety of invented traditions. . . . Today scholars are more concerned than ever before about 'how knowledge is arrived at' (302:76–77) and about how the past is perceived" (Krech 1991, p. 363, quoting Dening 1988, p. 75; Keesing 1990, p. 159; Price 1983, p. 241; and Tomkins 1986, p. 302).

10. Those others are indicated in my encyclopedia article in the preceding section.

11. Also, "In the 1970s, a more advanced tomography technique was developed by Michael Phelps and Edward Hoffman, a pair of biophysicists from the UCLA School of Medicine. Their technique, called positron emission tomography (PET) . . ." (Travers and Muhr 1994).

12. From http://www.conference-cast.com/snm/2001/biography.htm, last accessed March 22, 2003.

13. Dr. Michel M. Ter-Pogossian passed away on June 19, 1996.

14. See Bruno Latour's work for examples and on analysis of the history of science as a war game (Latour 1987; Latour 1988) Some alternate histories of medical sciences can be found in Cartwright (1995), Kaplan (1983), and Koch (1990). Anthropologist Michael Fischer has begun characterizing the poetics of scientific autobiographical discourse (Fischer 1995).

15. His coworkers in this tinkering include Nizar Mullani, John Hood, Jerome Cox, and Don Snyder.

16. Hawkins and Miller (1978), Huang and Veech (1982), Sacks et al. (1983). This controversy was made public with Fox (1984).

17. Gjedde and Kuwabara (1993), and Nelson et al. (1985).

18. Powers and Raichle (1985), Raichle (1985), and Wagner (1985).

19. Fluorine-18 is also considered a physiological radionuclide because it can easily substitute for hydrogen.

20. Hammersmith was the first for medical use, but St. Louis was the first as a direct part of a medical school.

21. Partially quoted earlier.

Chapter 3

1. Authorship actually varies quite a bit by discipline. Sometimes a listing as the last author is presumed to be a privilege. In some cases, the authors are listed alphabetically (see Biagioli et al. 1994; Galison 1997; and Traweek 1988).

2. The introduction of physical scientists into the medical world is modifying clinical practice in various ways. The most striking change lies in the introduction of new responsibilities and modifications in the distribution of existing ones to a point that physicists now share the physician's role in many diagnostic, therapeutic, and rehabilitation processes. Thus, after some 40 years of outstanding progress with brilliant contributions, the physicist is no longer considered a "back room boy," unknown to the patient and regarded to many clinicians as just another paramedic accessory. The introduction of physicists and technological innovations in medicine has been shown to have also a more direct impact on clinical practice. The clinicians themselves are involved in every step of the innovation process in the creation of new methods and devices and their diffusion at a professional level (Franconi 1983, p. 1).

3. These problems remain unresolved at the level of clinical trials in general. See Marks 1997 and also Rosser 1994.

4. I have adapted this quotation from a broader argument found in Sue V. Rosser's comprehensive review essay of androcentric bias in psychiatry. Rosser's entire book, a series of review essays on clinical research and treatment for women in the United States, is relevant to the questions I am raising regarding producing medical population data.

5. Robins (1990) has provided a history of epidemiological sampling for psychiatric illness. He emphasized the difficulty of accounting for minority groups because if they are counted at all, they often are oversampled, leading to an overestimation of their difference from the majority group.

6. That would also imply that this book was produced by a potentially abnormal "caffeinated" mind.

7. A different but telling example was cited by David Hull regarding blood types (A, B, O) in indigenous populations: "A is common in Europe, Scandinavia, Japan and Australia, rare in Africa, totally absent in South America. B is common in Asia, Africa, parts of Europe, absent everywhere else. O is prevalent in North and South America, fairly common in Africa, rare elsewhere" (Hull 1992, p. 59).

8. "All PET studies — whether while resting or doing a specific task — are acti-

vation studies because the brain continues to work even during nonspecific stimulation during resting" (Metter 1991).

9. The difficulty of actually imaging schizophrenic patients while they are hallucinating has been noted as a confounder. The typical imaged schizophrenic patient is selected for being able to submit to a lengthy and delicate scan procedure (see, e.g., Metz 1989).

10. See Frith (1991), especially the discussion following the article (pp. 191–196), for a discussion of some of these issues.

11. Another researcher commented that "it must be assumed that all individuals use similar cognitive processes during the task. This is not always the case" (Mazziotta et al. 1982; Metter 1991).

12. Another researcher begins an article entitled "Exploring the Mind with Dynamic Imaging" similarly: "Substantial evidence supports the hypothesis that the human brain is structurally and functionally modular" (Raichle 1990).

13. The only PET studies as of 1994 that examined the issue of language difference directly were done at McGill University in Montreal, Canada. The group examined English with French as a fluent second language and decided: "We find no evidence . . . that a language learned later in life is represented [in the brain] differently from the native language" (Editorial 1995; Klein et al. 1994; Klein et al. 1995). However, see also the Kanji studies of Sakurai et al. 1992.

14. "'If modules exist, then . . . double dissociations are a relatively reliable way of uncovering them. Double dissociations do exist. Therefore modules exist.' Presented in this form the logical fallacy is obvious" (Uttal 2001, p. 248).

15. See also Kosslyn (1994), Szasz (1996), and Wilson (1998).

16. Danziger (1990a) provides a history of task design in different psychological schools.

17. Raven's test is used by individual psychologists as a measure of general IQ.

18. See Saha, MacIntyre, and Go 1992; Wolf 1981b). Gallium-68, bromine-75, rubidium-82, and copper-62 can be produced without a cyclotron, using a "generator." Other articles list the half-life of oxygen-15 as 2.04 minutes (Welch and Kilbourn 1984).

19. For most PET researchers, the cyclotron is currently a black box: Its production process is standardized and automated, and the cyclotron is not something that generates errors. In fact, at most research institutions, one should not mess with the cyclotron.

20. Fluorine-18 can be and has been produced regionally and distributed to hospitals, but this limits the kinds of imaging that can be done with PET.

21. There is no consensus over what to actually call the labeled molecule. The Positron Emission Panel of the Council of Scientific Affairs of the American Medical Association prefers *labeled tracer* as the most accurate term (Council on Scientific Affairs Reports 1988). There has been a long debate over whether *radiopharmaceutical* is proper in the case of nuclear medicine. Some researchers have argued against this term because "the quantities of chemicals (both radioactive and nonradioactive) used in these agents are so minuscule that they fall below the level of immunoresponsiveness" and are therefore not pharmaceuti-

cals or "drugs" (Subramanian 1974). These definitional battles are not trivial, because pharmaceuticals are regulated quite differently from radiodiagnostic agents, (International Atomic Energy Agency 1971). This definition currently seems to be moot, however, because the Food and Drug Administration (FDA) continues to exercise jurisdiction over PET tracers in the United States (Levine and Abel 1990; Siegel 1981).

22. The story usually includes an anecdote about von Hevesy using this radioactive lead to prove that his landlady reused leftover meat in the hash she served later in the week (Brucer 1978).

23. From the chemist's perspective, choosing the right molecule to label is *the* critical element of PET. Edward Hoffman said, "You know, the heart of the whole thing is chemistry. I always had the faith that if the right application isn't here now, some young chemist is probably going to learn to synthesize the right thing, probably with fluorine-18, and it will be very important. Well, we have FDG, but not too many more things!"

The challenge for the chemist is to figure out how to convince a radioisotope to properly bind to the molecule, which involves making sure that in the process, the solution produced is relatively pure (free from other radiolabeled substances) and retains high enough (radio)activity so that the tracer will be detectable. Of course, the solution injected into the patient is mostly nonradioactive; the labeled molecule is only a tiny percentage of it, a *trace* amount.

For some molecules, such as oxygen gas (O_2) or carbon monoxide (CO), the production process is quite straightforward. For others, like FDG, the process involves a lot of precise, hands-on work. Currently, an entire branch of PET work concerns labeling new molecules, drugs in particular, and is the subject of many doctoral dissertations. Unfortunately, this field is also extremely labor intensive without clear signs of rewards. Many years are often invested in these attempts, and often they are completely unsuccessful, as described by one researcher:

> I have seen researchers spend years trying to develop a specific ligand [a radiotracer] and do the modeling work, and then the monkey work [i.e., testing it on an animal], and everything, trying to get the ligand into humans. The upshot was that if they picked the wrong tracer, five years or more of work basically goes to nothing because of something that couldn't have been foreseen.

The labeling process takes place in "hot labs" ("hot" for the radioactivity), where chemists work behind heavy shields and under hoods with prosthetic arms. One of their primary concerns is radiation dose, which is measured via badges or rings (rings because the isotope is often handled by hand, exposing the fingers more than the rest of the body). As the government has set strict yearly and lifetime dose limits and exceeding these limits means having to stay out of the lab for months at a time, the chemists have to balance carefully exposure with experience.

Computers have also joined the team of chemists. Since the late 1980s, some researchers spend almost all of their time in front of a monitor instead of in the lab. Using high-speed graphics workstations, they take the results of X-ray crystallography and model the physical structure of the molecule so as to measure better and then predict which isotopes will successfully bind and which will not. Ideally, this process saves years of trial and error. One chemical modeler explained that the cost of modeling was that one had to more or less give up the lab. Like good lab hands, he explained, "you have to be constantly working with the computer, programming, playing with it, getting to know its idiosyncrasies, in order to get good results. If you are away too long, you forget."

24. Maximum positron ranges: carbon-11 = 4.1 mm; nitrogen-13 = 5.1 mm; oxygen-15 = 7.3 mm; fluorine-18 = 2.4 mm.

25. The patient lies down on a movable table, and his or her head is held firmly in place. Because the slightest head movement can result in a blurry scan, keeping the head steady is an important task. Head holders are often designed specifically for each subject. In some institutions, a special kind of thermoplastic mask is molded to subjects' faces, and this is affixed to the bed and can be kept aligned. (Kearfott et al. 1984). For information on other head holders and positioning systems, see Kingsley et al. (1980), Mazziotta et al. (1982), Vanier et al. (1985).

For subjects who must remain immobile for 30 minutes to an hour, some technicians have come up with innovative ways of keeping them comfortable, such as placing an intravenous fluids bag, filled with water, under their head or playing music in the background. Institutions have reported that they often manually examine images for signs of head movement: "Any pair of PET studies that generate characteristic crescent-shaped areas of positive or negative changes are discarded without further processing" (Mintun et al. 1989).

Some of the technicians I talked with reported that between 1980 and the early 1990s, they were being slowly automated out of their jobs. Initially they not only kept the subject comfortable, monitored the scanner, and withdrew blood samples, but also performed much of the image analysis on the data, before sending it on to the researchers. Two trends intervened to make the technicians' jobs more boring. First, as computers became more powerful and affordable and graphics workstations fit onto desktops, researchers created teams of programmers to process and reprocess the raw radioactive data themselves. Second, commercial programs appeared that black-boxed many of the processing algorithms, allowing researchers to buy their image-processing software off the shelf. Injection is thus also becoming more and more black-boxed.

26. Different kinds of scintillation crystals include sodium iodide (NaI), bismuth germanate (BGO), and cesium flouride (CsF). Each of these crystals is quite dense, and the tightly packed atoms are thus better able to stop the gamma rays than the body is. Each gamma ray enters the crystal and begins to run into atoms dislodging electrons while losing energy. As each electron returns to its normal energy state, it releases energy in the form of a photon of light. This process is called scintillation. Crystals also have different resolution times, which refer to how discriminating the crystal is between two different gamma rays in time. Some crystals, such as CsF, for example, are so fast that they can distinguish not only coincidence windows but also the time between the arrival of each of the two gamma rays. This allows the scanner to interpret *where* the positron was along the line between the two detectors. This is known as time-

of-flight information, and time-of-flight PET scanners have been developed on this principle (Yamamoto et al. 1983; Yamamoto et al. 1982; Zimmerman 1988).

27. In conventional nuclear medicine, radioisotope decay results in gamma rays of varying and usually lesser intensity, and these rays are random in their directions. To assess their point of origin, collimators were developed, which were dense shields arranged such that only gamma rays traveling in one direction could get past them. Gamma rays traveling at angles would hit the collimators and be absorbed (see figure 3.5a). Collimators thus made localization possible at the cost of sensitivity: "Though you had a good idea of where the gamma rays were coming from, very few of them were ever counted. Thus, a higher dose of radioactivity would be needed to produce enough counts" (Wilson 1988).

Because the gamma rays from positron emitters come in pairs traveling in opposite directions, it is possible to perform "electronic collimation" by assuming that if two detectors register gamma ray hits at almost exactly the same time, then there most probably was positron decay along the line between the two detectors (Phelps et al. 1975).

In a PET scanner, then, detectors are arranged in a ring around the subject — often more than one ring (or hexagon). Each of these detectors is wired together so that near-simultaneous hits (within, e.g., 20 nanoseconds) can be registered, and the three-dimensional line between them can be passed on to the next stage of the imaging process.

The architecture of the PET scanner determines the sampling it is able to achieve. Sampling is the relative ability of the detectors to capture as much information as possible within the field of view. More detectors and smaller detectors contribute to better sampling and also better resolution (the size of each volume area being sampled). Both sampling and resolution tend to vary between the center and the edge of the field of view.

Although the principles remained the same between 1974 and 1994, some researchers have described PET scanners as fitting into three generations: The first generation consisted of single-ring scanners and began with the PETT series at Washington University in the early 1970s. The second generation consisted of multislice scanners and new types of crystal detectors and began in the early 1980s. The third generation of scanners became more complex and more practical for clinical use and began in the mid-1980s. See Koeppe and Hutchins (1992) for a complete review of these generations.

28. It is possible to view the data temporally to look for time-course information. Usually, however, the time-course data do not have enough counts (enough radioactivity) per time segment to produce an accurate picture. Even in this case, to get any picture at all, some time segment must be condensed into a state.

29. In an interview, Henry Wagner described for me the meaning of *functional* in this case:

A researcher named Shigekoto Kaihara is the one who coined the term *functional image*. That then subsequently got translated into what is called parametric imaging, but that guy, actually in a paper that he published in

195

1968 here at Johns Hopkins, when he was a trainee, the whole paper was in the title. It said, "the construction of a functional image from rate constants." He took rate constants, spatial measurements, and instead of putting distribution in space, he displayed the distribution of the rate constant and called it a functional image. So that is the only way you can handle that much quantitative data. Plus it has the additional advantage of relating it to space, so it relates space and time. The essence of physiology is time.

30. PET experiments are founded on the assumption that the flow of these molecules is different in different regions of the brain and that this difference is related to the activity of that part of the brain. Brain activations are fast biochemical and biophysical activity increases. The bulk of these fast changes occur in the synaptic regions. The energy demands are therefore the highest in synaptic regions when the brain activates. The extra demands on glucose and oxygen also result in increases of the regional cerebral blood flow (Seitz and Roland 1992).

Another assumption of PET is that the regions of the brain that show these differences are not necessarily the regions of the brain delineated by anatomists. John Mazziotta, neuroanatomist and neurologist at the University of California, Los Angeles, declared this assumption in an editorial: "A basic premise that must be discarded is that structural and functional anatomy are equivalent" (Mazziotta 1984). The concept of "function" that Mazziotta invoked is internal to the PET experiment: A study that shows a certain area of the brain "lighting up" in response to a verb-generation task refers to the area corresponding to the "verb generation" function, regardless of whether this area corresponds to a nicely delineated anatomical structure (Petersen et al. 1989). The PET image may show a "circuit" of areas that together comprise the "function" (Begley 1991; Raichle 1994b).

A related but different concept of function refers back to Shigekoto Kaihara's article, "The Construction of a Functional Image from Spatially Localized Rate Constants Obtained from Serial Camera and Rectilinear Scanner Data." This concept is also internal to the imaging experiment. A "functional image" in Kaihara's sense is one in which each pixel corresponds to the value of a mathematical function that describes the rate of flow of the molecule in that anatomical area. In some PET images, for example, red areas mean that those areas of the brain had a flow rate twice that of blue areas. "In a sense, the scanning image may be thought of as a map of regional function" (Kaihara et al. 1969).

31. His technical discussion reveals the true difficulty faced in standardizing brains:

> As we discussed above, SPM [uses the brains from the MNI for its templates. SPM99b uses the MNI average of 152 scans, and SPM96 uses the scan data from the individual brain that has been scanned many times. . . . This means that the Talairach atlas is not exactly accurate for interpreting coordinates from SPM analyses, if (as is almost always the case) the scans have been spatially normalized (coregistered) to the SPM 99 or SPM 96 template. This can be a problem, as, to my knowledge, there is currently

no published MNI atlas, defining Brodmann's areas on the MNI brain. In contrast there is extensive information on Brodmann's areas for the Talairach atlas. . . . However, the SPM authors have referred to the coordinates from SPM96,99 analyses (matched to the MNI brain) as being "in Talairach space". . . . By this they mean that the coordinates are reported in terms of the system that Talairach developed, with coordinate 0,0,0 being at the anterior commissure (AC), and with the anterior/posterior commissural line (AC/PC line) defining the plane where z = 0. (In fact the AC is not exactly at 0,0,0 in the MNI brain, but about 4mm below — see the 152 T1 average brain in the canonical directory). However, they do not mean by this that the coordinates match the brain in the Talairach atlas, because this is not precisely the case."

After providing some transformations himself, he concludes:

Other methods that you can use to work out where your activation is are: (1) Use the SPM 99 and 96 overlay displays to show you the activations on the MNI brain. If you know your anatomy well, or can see the equivalent structures in the Talairach atlas, then you may know where your activation is. Unfortunately, outside the primary sensorimotor cortices, the relation of functional areas to sulcal anatomy can be very variable; (2) Use the Talairach atlas, and try by eye to take into account the difference in brain size (given that the differences are relatively small). Obviously this can be inaccurate, and it is very difficult to standardize across labs.

32. Automatically or semiautomatically.

33. See Valentino (1991) for a comprehensive review of mapping and registering strategies. See also Mazziotta and Koslow (1987) for a survey of different institutional methods. Specific methods include those explicated by Bajcsy et al. (1983), Fox et al. (1985), and Mazziotta et al. (1991).

34. Tracer-kinetic modeling is both a unique strength of PET and its most complicated weakness. When done carefully, and assuming the assumptions hold, modeling allows PET to produce truly quantitative information about the precise amount of the molecule in each region of the brain. Without modeling, only relative differences and relative changes are possible to measure. Whether absolute quantitation is necessary or even valuable has been the subject of debate for decades (Strother et al. 1991). Again, this debate is one of paradigms with implication for the meaning of the data. Does it matter, for instance, if the whole brain is less active in some subjects or during some activities, or do only relative differences between different regions matter?

To reduce the technical complexity of this stage, I have moved a discussion of biomathematics to this note. This step consists in turning the reconstructed matrix of counts, the data set, into the actual physiological information. In 1981, Barbara Croft defined the difference between what she called "direct functional imaging, in which images of a particular radiopharmaceutical distribution are used by themselves," and "indirect functional imaging, in which the images are formed by mathematical manipulation" (Croft 1981). The reconstructed data set represents a direct functional image at this point, the amount of radioactive material that was present in each area of the brain during the period of the scan. Because the relationship between the isotope and the brain action is quite complex, as noted earlier, the data require mathematical manipulation. Croft called these indirect functional images "parametric."

> In order to convert these data to meaningful information such as is implied by the processes listed above or any other than can be studied by PET, a model that allows the determination of the particular process, e.g., glucose metabolism, is required. This is the essence of the PET method and sets it apart from methods whose primary purpose is imaging. (Wolf 1981a)

The kinds of parametric scans can be divided into two types: accumulation and flow, with variances to be discussed later. Accumulation scans are like iodine scans in the thyroid; a tracer is introduced that flows through the body and is "trapped" in particular areas. Studies of cancer metastases work on this principle. FDG, for example, travels like glucose across the blood–brain barrier and into cells, where, because it is not glucose, it goes through only some of the reactions glucose does. It stops reacting before it gets kicked back out of the cell. Therefore, the accumulation of FDG in cells represents a percentage of the glucose activity that cell during the period of uptake. In quantitative FDG studies, blood samples are taken at 15 seconds, 30 seconds, 60 seconds, 2 minutes, and so on, to measure the amount of radioactivity in the blood at each time. This produces a time-activity curve that allows an estimate of the actual amount of FDG glucose trapped in each area of the brain at each point in time. Without this blood sampling, only the relative amounts of FDG activity can be measured (i.e., activity in frontal lobes relative to activity in the cerebellum).

Of course, this trapping process of FDG in the cells is metabolically complicated. There are many variables to consider in using the data set of counts to figure out how much activity was going on in each region of the brain. What is ultimately measured is the average rate of accumulation of FDG over a period of time.

Flow studies are similar conceptually: During a 2-minute oxygen scan, for instance, the radioactive blood is circulating through the brain. Areas with more activity are assumed to have increased flow. Thus, more blood is present to be counted. Again, there are models of the relation between flow and activity, but the final result is a data set of the rate of flow.

FDG and oxygen are the more simple kinds of studies. In neurotransmitter studies, not only must the amount of the labeled tracer be estimated for each area but the reactions by the brain to the tracer must also be estimated. See Kilbourn and Zalutsky (1985) for an excellent technical overview of receptor imaging with PET. As a dopamine agonist arrives and binds to dopamine receptors, possible reactions include more or less dopamine becoming available, more receptors, increased receptivity of the receptors, and increased or decreased activity in other neurotransmitters. The actual design of models, testing, and estimation of parameters is a long and complicated process. One postdoctoral researcher described his experience with kinetic modeling:

> To study certain topics, some of us are using models to calculate different kinds of parameters, like disassociation constants and so on. These kinds

of things we have to do when we use a new ligand, just to define the ligand. For example, the ligand that I am working [on] now is for opiate receptors. First, I have to see how specific the binding is: Does the ligand bind just to the opiate receptors I am interested in, or does it also bind to other kinds of receptors? The next step will be to define the compartmental model: the association and disassociation constants, the transport wave over the blood–brain barrier back and forth.

See Carson (1986) on parameter estimations and Huang and Phelps (1986) on the principles of tracer kinetic modeling.

35. This project involves securing a number of brains of deceased people, freezing them in the skull, and then slicing them with a microcryotome, producing high-resolution photographic images of micron-level detail. An entire database of cells, neurons, and so forth can be built up in this process. Variability is accounted for by using many brains instead of just one.

36. Per Roland devotes the last chapter (the final 10 of 600 pages) to potential problems deriving from variability issues. In addition to functional-anatomical variability, tracer-related variability, data normalization and transformation variability, and institutional variability are all significant concerns (Roland 1993). Ford et al. surveyed these concerns and offered this: "Because of the complexity of the data collected and the questions of interest, the extent to which these problems truly influence biological conclusions is difficult to assess. This uncertainty is in itself one of the major issues facing this area of research" (Ford et al. 1991, p. A94).

37. See especially Pawlik (1988), and Pawlik (1991).

38. Kosslyn (1989) commented that most visual displays make poor use of color. On color coding in PET, see especially Dr. Wagner's "Color in Nuclear Medicine: Contribution or Camouflage?" which argues in favor of the American adoption of pseudo-color scales. He notes: "The colors we instruct the computer to assign . . . are arbitrary only in the sense that not all of us have as yet agreed on what they mean. Once we agree on a color code and become practiced in it, the issue of arbitrariness disappears and the result is shared experience and a new language with which we can communicate more effectively" (Wagner 1974).

39. See also Jardine (1992).

40. I am currently investigating the history of conventions by which extremes are chosen for visual display and by which differences among types are emphasized over variability within types — the usefulness of typing in this way at all.

41. See Nelkin and Tancredi (1989) for a discussion of the problem of false-positives in experimental research. See also Ford (1983) and Rapoport (1991) for discussions of the implications of type I and II errors.

42. In another set of images on the facing page, the scans are labeled *normals* and *schizophrenics* illustrating the difficulty of keeping these labels clear. The volunteers for this study are perhaps better described as normal subjects with no history of psychiatric diagnosis (the normals) and normal subjects with no history of psychiatric diagnosis other than schizophrenia (the schizophrenics).

43. See Brodie et al. (1983), Delisi and Buchsbaum (1986), Ford et al. (1991), Phelps and Mazziotta (1985), and Volkow and Wolf (1991).

44. The most sustained attack on these anti-psychiatrists (including a fantasy trial in which they are condemned by parents of those with mental illness) was by Torrey (1983).

45. See Faulstich and Sullivan (1991). Metz (1989) provides a conceptual and technical critique of the psychiatric diagnosis with PET.

46. Another train of reasoning is the "modeling critique" defined by Charlton (1990) and based on Bernard's critique of averages in physiology. The production of explicatory images risks producing an "average schizophrenic" who is "perhaps more of a mythical beast than the so-called 'classic cases' of other branches of medicine" (p. 4). Averages also condense into a steady state what is in fact a variable in time, a pulsatile phenomenon.

47. Consider, for example, the following statements culled from contemporary neuroscience: "Today, of course, there is hardly a respectable neuroscientist alive who thinks the mind exists apart from the functions of the physical brain and body" (Montgomery 1989, p. 67). Gazzaniga (1989) commented on the "organization of the human brain" in *Science*: "An emerging view is that the brain is structurally and functionally organized into discrete units or 'modules' and that these components interact to produce mental activities" (p. 947). Le-Vay (1993) stated that even though culture and environment might be opposed to genetics, all fall under biology: "Thinking about the mind in biological terms is not the same thing as believing that all mental states are genetically determined, since even environmental and cultural influences on the mind operate through biological mechanisms."

48. See especially Metz (1989), in which difficulties with PET are highlighted and the author calls for focusing on PET-distinguished groups.

Chapter 4

1. The first CT scan of a patient was performed in 1971 by EMI. Kevles (1997) discussed the rapidity with which CT entered the medical and popular imagination, with five contracts awarded during 1972. Nonetheless, Kevles also notes that "the first CT images were a puzzle to the physicians and surgeons who would be expected to use them (Vanoverschelde et al. 1993). Ledley [American inventor of a CT scanner] recalls that he felt obliged in 1976 to publish his own atlas to teach radiologists how to see the images his ACTA produced" (p. 162).

2. See, for example, Andreasen (1984) and Kuhar (1990).

3. Quoted in Froehlich (1987, p. 17).

4. Other researchers have commented on the difficulties of drawing conclusions from the newest machines with the best resolution. Because there are no other devices capable of generating comparable data, they have no way of knowing what it is that they are seeing.

5. As mentioned before, this demand for programmatic clarity is part of the court system. It is also at the basis of U.S. malpractice claims resulting in defensive medicine, wherein deviation from standardized medical protocol is avoided

for fear of lawsuits. See Konner (1993) for an analysis of this system and alternatives to it.

6. Shelton and Weinberger (1986) reviewed "more than 100 CT studies investigating brain abnormalities in schizophrenia. . . . Most of these studies (75%) have reported enlarged lateral ventricles even though fewer than 10% of the CT scans have been interpreted as abnormal by a clinical neuroradiologist . . . this emphasizes the subtlety of the changes noted in schizophrenia" (cited in Shenton et al. 1997, p. 299). Shenton et al. reviewed sixty-seven MRI studies as well as the CT studies and discovered a variety of divergent findings. Ventricle enlargement in particular was discussed as being correlated with schizophrenia in twenty-seven of thirty-seven studies that looked at it, but some of those included significant enlargement only in men (two studies) or only in women (two studies). In addition, they began their discussion noting that "enlarged lateral ventricles are not, however, specific to schizophrenia as there are many other disorders such as Alzheimer's disease and Huntington's chorea that can result in enlarged lateral ventricles" (p. 380).

7. The decision in *Daubert* v. *Merrell Dow Pharmaceuticals, Inc.* (113 S. Ct. 2786 1993) and its ramifications go beyond the narrow considerations discussed in this book. *Daubert* changed the focus of admission of scientific testimony from a "general acceptance" test, including peer review, to one in which the trial judge evaluates expert scientific testimony at the outset, considering many issues such as validation, testability, falsifiability, and peer review. See Jasanoff (1995) for an excellent analysis of the changing legal and scientific landscape in the wake of *Daubert*.

8. Caught here is the sublime dilemma of brain imaging. The researcher finds it almost impossible to argue that the yellow blob or any other "abnormality" might mean that the person is "completely normal."

9. Paul MacLean has been quoted as saying, "One of the worst things in the world is to be 'discovered' by the popular media" (Harrington 1992).

10. Michael (1994).

11. I have not figured out why Hatfield reported 12 men and 2 women whereas Begley reported 13 men and 4 women.

12. For an illuminating look at popular turn-of-the-nineteenth-century futurism surrounding X-rays, see Knight (1986).

Chapter 5

1. *Frame* is used here to denote the whole arrangement of images and captions, and its positioning in an article on mapping the brain, in *Newsweek*, oriented toward an educated audience. See, for example, Barthes (1968), Dumit (1995a), Haraway (1991), and Hartouni (1992) on framing and audience.

2. Other influences include books, magazines, television, the advice of our doctors, and reported experiences of our friends.

3. See, for example, Huff (1954), which focuses primarily on the visual persuasiveness of certain kinds of graph presentations.

4. Nelson Goodman's elegant "Seven Strictures on Similarity" offers a con-

trary perspective in which "circumstances alter similarities" (Goodman 1992, p. 21)

5. She also describes the *New Yorker* magazine cartoons:

> which in a few drawn lines capture layers of nuance. Moreover, such images often carry profound cultural meaning or suggest stories told with wit and intelligence through symbolism or metaphor. Paralleling the process of perception itself, such images reveal a contempt for indiscriminate attention and for superfluous detail; they eschew the irrelevant and reveal the pattern that emerges only from essential characteristics in synchrony. (Barry 1997, p. 77)

6. *Being caught* should not be confused with *believing*. Anthropology has a long history of critiquing the concept of belief, as if culture could be reduced to false knowledge or reasonable mistakes about the world (Good 1994); see also Douglas 1966; Douglas and Hull 1992; and Levi-Strauss 1966)

7. Functional magnetic resonance imaging (fMRI) is an adaptation of the software of MRI technology that shows images of blood flow rates in the brain similar to PET. See, for example, Kwong et al. (1992).

8. *Laypersons* is from *laity*, meaning "those before the cleric." "It is worth noting that 'layman' now means 'not a scientist' as before [it meant] 'not a cleric,' which suggests the same faith in the one kind of knowledge worth having" (Barzun 1964). See Ademuwagun (1979) for anthropological discussions of lay knowledge.

9. This can also be thought of as an "operational aesthetic" (Harris 1973), in which highbrow science is appropriated and played with by the masses. See also Dumit (2001).

10. Even if they are maintained unevenly (see Rapp 1999).

11. Delgado (1969) made similar pronouncements regarding brain waves and electrical stimulation via telemetry (see Dumit 1995a).

12. MEDLINE breaks down violence into the categories Aggression, Crime, Social Problems, Dangerous Behavior, and Domestic (though Domestic was added after 1990).

13. For instance, in an article, "Positron Emission Tomography and *in vivo* Brain Chemistry," Wagner stated:

> Perhaps it is not too far-fetched to believe that information about the chemistry of "toxic" emotions such as aggression and violence, can help control aggressive behavior, which seems to be built into human genes, and is encouraged by many human activities, from sports to watching television. Such emotions are reflected in measurable changes in the chemistry of the brain. Violence — both personal and cultural — may not be uncontrollable or inevitable, and perhaps one day will be regarded as aberrant behavior, a disease similar to other mental illness." (Wagner 1989, p. 130)

14. Jeffery (1994) contended that biological psychiatry and other biological research into behavior, together with the failure of prisons, implies the need for treatment of criminals or offering them a choice between prison and treatment. Current legal responses ignores the necessity of treating mentally dysfunctional

individuals. See also Monahan (1988), Sheard (1984), and Storr (1970) for evaluations of research on violence and aggression research. These reports urge a cautious approach especially to the problem of predicting violence and offer increasingly specific breakdowns of types and causes of violence. Menzies et al. (1985) argued that violence is too complex to study (i.e., it has too many causes and the term refers to too many different kinds of activities).

15. "'Ecstasy' Damages the Brain and Impairs Memory in Humans." Mathias, Robert. *NIDA Notes Research News*, vol. 14, no. 4, 1999. See http://www.nida.nih.gov/NIDA—Notes/ NNVol14N4/Ecstasy.html, accessed February 25, 2003. The text reads, in part:

> In the brain imaging study, researchers used positron emission tomography (PET) to take brain scans of 14 MDMA users who had not used any psychoactive drug, including MDMA, for at least 3 weeks. Brain images also were taken of 15 people who had never used MDMA. Both groups were similar in age and level of education and had comparable numbers of men and women.
>
> In people who had used MDMA, the PET images showed significant reductions in the number of serotonin transporters, the sites on neuron surfaces that reabsorb serotonin from the space between cells after it has completed its work. The lasting reduction of serotonin transporters occurred throughout the brain, and people who had used MDMA more often lost more serotonin transporters than those who had used the drug less.

16. Statement of the Director, National Institute on Drug Abuse, U.S. Senate Caucus on International Narcotics Control, July 25, 2000. See http://www.drugabuse.gov/Testimony/7-25-00Testimony.html, accessed March 22, 2003. The full caption reads:

> Figure 1 (right) shows the images of two human brains. Through the use of positron emission tomography (PET), we can actually see that the brain images on top belongs to an individual who has never used MDMA. The bottom images show the brain of an individual who had used MDMA heavily for an extended period, but was abstinent from drugs for at least three weeks prior to the study. Clearly the brain of the MDMA user on the bottom has been significantly altered. The specific parameter being measured is the brain's ability to bind the chemical neurotransmitter serotonin. Serotonin is critical to normal experiences of mood, emotion, pain, and a wide variety of other behaviors. On the figure, brighter colors reflect greater serotonin transporter binding; dull colors mean less binding capacity. This figure shows a decrease in the MDMA user's ability to remove this important neurotransmitter from the intercellular space, thereby amplifying its effects within the brain. This decrease lasts at least three weeks after the individual has stopped using MDMA.

17. It should be noted that the book *Rampage* (Wood 1985), on which the movie is based, does not mention PET scanning at all. It also has no pictures.

18. There is quite a lot of research on mental illness and violence. The legal

category in the United States is "dangerousness" (a danger to self or others can be grounds for involuntary commitment). Mestrovic and Cook (1986) and Monahan and Shah (1989) provide histories and evaluations of the dangerousness standard. Many researchers have argued that mental illness is actually *not* predictive of violence (Mulvey and Lidz 1984; Pollock 1990).

19. Movies and other media are often the direct route for new sciences like PET to enter the courtroom. Consider, for instance, the case of Barry Wayne McNamara, who on January 5, 1985, killed his parents, his sister, and his niece. When this case was brought to trial, McNamara's attorney, Santa Barbara Deputy Public Defender Michael McGrath thought his client was not sane and sought proof beyond psychiatrists diagnosing schizophrenia: "We know there was a trend in the law which is hostile to psychiatrists in the courtrooms. . . . What we needed was objective evidence." McGrath learned of PET scanning through a PBS television series, *The Brain*, and contacted Monte Buchsbaum at University at California, Irvine's Brain Imaging Center. Buchsbaum reported that McNamara received a life sentence and not the death penalty "partly, perhaps, because of the ameliorating circumstances of a brain which was not entirely normal" (Black 1989).

20. Contrary to this tendency, however, many researchers are worried that the ability to image successfully is more a triumph for science than for medicine. "We perceive victories for medicine because of the way we define victories. That more people are going to die of lung cancer this year than last is less important, apparently, than that we can see those cancers earlier with CT" (Ell 1988). Steven Selzer, commenting on this article, wondered "whether the mindset of medicine will shift, perhaps from the problems of individuals to those of populations" (Seltzer, 1988, p. 958). Robert Proctor's thesis on cancer as a social disease, one of the few diseases we know we can prevent by altering our daily practices, is worth reflecting on as such an alternate approach to medical intervention (Proctor 1991).

21. Merleau-Ponty (1964, p. 85), cited in Levin and Solomon (1990, p. 517).

22. Mauss (1985). See also Carrithers et al. (1985), Geertz (1973), Schweder and Bourne (1984), and Strathern (1992).

23. See, for example, Rhodes (1990) and Part III of Romanucci-Ross et al. (1991).

24. See Carrithers et al. 1985.

25. See Farquhar (1992), Manning and Fabrega (1973), Saunders (1989), Taussig (1991), and Taussig (1993).

26. See the works of Canguilhem (1988), Foucault et al. (1988), and Gilman (1988) especially; see also Terry (1989).

27. See Csordas (1990): "The body is not the object of study but the subject of culture." Culture entails science for us; therefore, our bodies have to take into account science.

28. I use *factoid* in the CNN sense of an apparently nonscientific, even pseudo-scientific claim. William Safire (1993), described many current definitions of *factoid*. He eventually declared that though he does not like it, CNN's constant use of the term means that CNN's notion of it will in the end prevail.

29. In chapters 4, 5, and 6 of this book, I am concerned with how facts are put together and disseminated, how authority and qualifications work together or are at odds with each other.

30. See Levi-Strauss (1963). See also Turkle (1984). "When one says in connection with totemism that certain animal species are chosen not because they are 'good to eat' but because they are 'good to think', one is no doubt disclosing an important truth. But it must not lead one to neglect the questions that then follow: why are some species 'better to think' than others; why is one pair of oppositions chosen over all the other possible pairs offered by nature; who thinks these pairs, when and how?" (Castoriadis 1984, p. 19).

31. See pages 244–249 of *Listening to Prozac* for Kramer's discussion of this.

32. On coming to identify with a group of like sufferers see Edgerton (1993), Rabinow (1992), and Rapp (1999). On the NAMI (National Alliance for the Mentally Ill), see Torrey (1983), among others. On the Twelve-Step movement, see Makela et al. (1996).

33. This is a rewording of Lutz's passage "We play with the terms of, but also ultimately satisfy, Western (cultural) common sense."

34. See especially, Browner and Press (1996), Rapp (1998), Shohat (1992), and Treichler (1991). This is further developed in Dumit (2000a).

35. Genes convey a future, a disposition for something to happen, and are in the modality of speed (Fortun 1998; Fortun 2001; Sunder Rajan 2002). Brains convey the present, a self, and are in the modality of infinite speed, the future now.

36. See Taylor (1998, pp. 19–20) on reassurance and bonding—psychological benefits provided by ultrasound (in addition to behavioral benefits)—through awareness of the fetus. These benefits all are seen as medical side effects. Other anthropologists have studied the varieties of experiencing the "real baby" through ultrasound (Mitchell and Georges 1998; Rapp 1998).

37. Brain research may also be used to reinforce stereotypes of race and sex, but in these situations, social identification is readily apparent when brain-types are produced and then affixed to the identification.

38. In Braude (1989), early spiritualists argued that they were able to function as mediums precisely to the extent that they could render their mind and body passive, letting the spirits speak through them. This is part of how women were able to turn the tables on assertions of their passivity: Men being active were therefore unsuited to be mediums.

39. On incorporations, see especially Crary and Kwinter (1992) and Diprose and Ferrell (1991).

40. The psychiatrist in this instance is using the PET scan to "therapeutically emplot" the patient as well. That is, by helping the patient to see mental illness as a physiological phenomenon, physiological intervention is also facilitated. See Good et al. (1994) and Mattingly (1994).

41. One researcher noted during our conversation that he should list this feeling of validation as a confounder in future PET studies of depressed patients.

42. See Post and Ballenger (1984), as cited in Kramer (1993, pp. 110–118, 334).

Chapter 6

1. An excellent historiographical inquiry into the history of descriptive psychopathology is provided by Berrios (1985). The journals *Psychological Medicine*, *Philosophy of Medicine and Biology*, and *Culture, Medicine and Psychiatry* provide forums for discussions of these issues.

2. Heath and Crabb (1993) surveyed research on depression in terms of a Western history of mind–body dualism and scientifically oriented biomedicine.

3. Starobinski (1990), for instance, historically investigated whether emotions are equated with bodily sensation in being opposed to cognition, or whether body consciousness is unitary, incorporating all of these "perceptions" into one process.

4. For cross-cultural investigations into emotion, see Kleinman and Good (1985), Levy (1984), Lutz (1988), Rosaldo (1980, 1984), and Schweder and LeVine (1984). On mental abnormalities, see Baer (1987), Johnson and Sargent (1990), and Romanucci-Ross et al. (1991).

5. For example, Kramer, in *Listening to Prozac*, compared length of grieving time in Greece with that in the United States (Kramer 1993, pp. 269–271).

6. Greimas and Fontanille (1993), see page 52 and the entire chapter. I do not think that they succeeded in their characterization of the passions, but they achieved the most comprehensive attempt to think through what is necessary to study them. MEDLINE breaks emotions down into *affect, anger, anxiety, bereavement, boredom, euphoria, fear, frustration, guilt, happiness, hate, hostility, jealousy, laughter,* and *love.* Of these, from 1990 to 1994, only *affect, fear,* and *anxiety* were listed as keywords in more than 1,000 articles.

7. See also James (1970 [1890]) and Solomon's analysis of James's theory of emotions with respect to anthropology (Solomon 1984).

8. Irigaray (1993) analyzed (Descartes's 1970) "Passions of the Soul," to recover "wonder" as the first of all passions.

9. This raises questions of the limits of thinking, because method acting involves bodily memory as much as cognitive skill.

10. On philosophical anthropology, see Blumenberg (1985), Buytendijk (1974), and Kant (1978). Also see Eccles (1989), Kosslyn and Koenig (1992), Luria (1973) and other neuroscientists on theorizing consciousness. It is probable, though, because of the challenge of theorizing emotions, that Mayberg must become a philosophical anthropologist earlier, and more thoroughly, at the beginning of her experiments, rather than in hindsight.

11. See Clarke and Dewhurst (1972) for a history of illustrations of such functional diagrams.

12. Berrios (1985) confirmed this: "The work on brain localization, for all its great importance to the development of neuropsychology, did not serve the emotions well as it concentrated on speech, perception and movement" (Meyer 1974; Tizard 1959, p. 745).

13. To go with artificial intelligence.

14. An extreme example of the computational metaphor of the mind is MacCormac's thesis of coevolution. In an article, he began by noting that computers

are similar to minds in many respects: storing data, recalling and manipulating it, and recognizing patterns:

> Although computers are faster . . . most of the differences between the two remain on the side of humans who have emotions, possess more creativity, and are intentional in many of their actions. . . . I presume the conceptual metaphor and propose the thesis that visual and auditory perceptual images serve as interactive devices between culture and the mind/brain, generating a coevolutionary process (biologic and cultural evolution)." (MacCormac 1989)

Emotions are explicitly excluded from this point on (even in considering art and language).

15. Pain and pleasure in neural network theory (itself painfully caught up in being the model for as well as modeled on the human brain) is translated into reward and punishment. In other words, they are also always understandable, reasonable, and purposeful (rewards and punishment teach neural nets how to rationally behave). In fact, the medical anthropological work of Byron Good and Jean Jackson on chronic pain explores the contradiction of pain of without purpose or understandability (Good et al. 1992; Jackson 1994, 2000).

16. These questions are elaborated in, for example, Fox (1994), Fox and Association of Social Anthropologists of the Commonwealth (1975), Konner (1982), and Kosslyn and Koenig (1992).

17. See Danziger (1990a), Kruger et al. (1987a), Kruger et al. (1987b), and Porter (1995). Phenomenologists should be glad to note that despite a long dry spell, they are once again being read by cutting-edge quantitative psychiatric and neurological researchers.

18. Heidegger (1962). Of course, Heidegger also privileged the mood (?) of caring, which is as much a social relation as a neurological state.

19. These metaphors are elaborated in Ronell (1989), Shannon and Weaver (1962), Wiener (1948), and Wiener and Schade (1965).

20. Though why they are not considered as important in cognitive psychology is a good question. For a summary critique of neurotransmitters as being ever more numerous and therefore too complex to model, see Charlton (1990).

21. PET studies of memory include those by Fazio et al. (1992) and Heiss et al. (1992). Perani et al. (1992) argued that PET demonstrates the clusters of cerebral areas associated with different memory function components, "in agreement with 'neural network' models of the neural basis of cognition, according to which complex functions are subserved by multiple interconnected cortical and subcortical structures" (p. 903).

22. An area related to regulation is coordination. How do all of these highly specialized circuits work together? Kosslyn, in *Wet Mind*, posited (in the final 20 pages) a "decider" circuit that weighs each decision, taking into account emotional weight. Other researchers use different metaphors:

> [Steven E.] Peterson favors "a localized region or a small number of localized regions," where perceptions, memories and intentions are inte-

grated. Goldman-Rakic is leaning toward a nonhierarchical model in which "separate but equal partners are interconnected, communicating with each other." (Horgan 1993)

23. I hesitate to use this metaphor as current, because it implies that other metaphors are outdated. This book has been trying to show that there are many, often contradictory, metaphors alive at the same time, distributed unevenly.

24. PET is marketed to the NIH, for instance, rather than health maintenance organizations—so far. On the congressional declaration of the 1990s as the Decade of the Brain, see Ackerman (1992).

25. See, for example, Haraway (1991), Hartouni (1991), Martin (1990), Rapp (1998), and Triechler (1999).

Bibliography

Ackerman, Sandra. *Discovering the Brain*. Washington, D.C.: National Academy Press, 1992.

Ademuwagun, Z. A. *African Therapeutic Systems*. Los Angeles: Crossroads Press, 1979.

Ader, Mary. "Investigational Treatments: Coverage, Controversy, and Consensus." *Annals of Health Law* 5 (1996): 45–61.

Althusser, Louis. *Essays on Ideology*. London: Verso, 1984, 1976.

Andreasen, Nancy C. *The Broken Brain: The Biological Revolution in Psychiatry*. New York: Harper & Row, 1984.

———. "Linking Mind and Brain in the Study of Mental Illnesses: A Project for a Scientific Psychopathology." *Science* 275, no. 5306 (1997): 1586–1593.

———. *Brave New Brain: Conquering Mental Illness in the Era of the Genome*. Oxford, New York: Oxford University Press, 2001.

Andreasen, Nancy C., ed. *Brain Imaging: Applications in Psychiatry*. Washington, D.C.: American Psychiatric Press, 1989.

Appadurai, Arjun. "Introduction: Commodities and the Politics of Value." In *The Social Life of Things: Commodities in Cultural Perspective*, ed., Arjun Appadurai, pp. 3–63. Cambridge: Cambridge University Press, 1986.

Ashmore, Malcolm. *The Reflexive Thesis: Wrighting Sociology of Scientific Knowledge*. Chicago: University of Chicago Press, 1989.

Baer, Hans A., ed. *Encounters with Biomedicine: Case Studies in Medical Anthropology*, Health, Society, and Culture; vol. 1. New York: Gordon and Breach Science Publishers, 1987.

Bajcsy, R., R. Lieberson, and M. Reivich. "A Computerized System for the Elastic Matching of Deformed Radiographic Images to Idealized Atlas Images." *Journal of Computer Assisted Tomography* 7, no. 4 (1983): 618–625.

Barry, Ann Marie. *Visual Intelligence: Perception, Image, and Manipulation in Visual Communication*. Albany: State University of New York Press, 1997.

Barthes, Roland. *Elements of Semiology*. Translated by Annette Laver and Colin Smith. New York: Hill and Wang, 1968.

———. *The Fashion System*. Translated by Matthew Ward and Richard Howard. New York: Hill and Wang, 1983.

———. *Criticism and Truth*. Minneapolis: University of Minnesota Press, 1987.

———. *Semiotic Challenge*. Translated by Richard Howard. New York: Farrar, Strauss and Giroux, 1988.

Barzun, Jacques. *Science: The Glorious Entertainment*. New York: Harper & Row, 1964.

Beaulieu, Anne E. "The Space Inside the Skull: Digital Representations, Brain Mapping and Cognitive Neuroscience in the Decade of the Brain." Amsterdam: University of Amsterdam, 2000.

Becker, Anne E. *Body, Self, and Society: The View from Fiji*. Philadelphia: University of Pennsylvania Press, 1995.

Begley, Sharon. "Thinking Looks Like This: PET Scans Show the Brain Recalling and Cogitating. (Positron Emission Tomography)." *Newsweek* 118, no. 22 (1991): 67(1).

———. "Mapping the Brain." *Newsweek* (1992): April 20, 66(5).

———. "Gray Matters: New Brain-Scanning Technologies Show Differences Between Men and Women." *Newsweek* (1995): March 27, 48(7).

Bergson, Henri. *Matter and Memory*. New York: Zone Books, 1988.

Berrios, G. E. "The Psychopathology of Affectivity: Conceptual and Historical Aspects." *Psychological Medicine* 15 (1985): 745–758.

Biagioli, Mario, Roddey Reid, and Sharon Traweek, eds. *Located Knowledges: Intersections between Cultural, Gender and Science Studies* (Special Issue of *Configurations*, vol. 2, no. 1). Baltimore: Johns Hopkins University Press, 1994.

Black, Randall. "What's On Your Client's Mind? PET Scans of Brain Can Let You Look." *UCI Journal* Jan.–Feb. (1989): 5.

Blumenberg, Hans. *Work on Myth*. Studies in Contemporary German Social Thought. Cambridge, Mass.: MIT Press, 1985.

Blumenthal, Dale. "Image Processing Advanced Techniques Enable Scientists to Pursue New Studies." *NIH Record* 24, no. 8 (1982): 11.

Bourdieu, Pierre. "The Specificity of the Scientific Field and the Social Conditions of the Progress of Reason." *Social Science Information* 14, no. 6 (1975): 19–57.

———. *In Other Words: Essays Towards a Reflexive Sociology*. Translated by Matthew Adamson. Stanford, Calif.: Stanford University Press, 1990.

Boyle, Mary. *Schizophrenia: A Scientific Delusion?* London: Routledge, 1990.

Braude, Ann. *Radical Spirits: Spiritualism and Women's Rights in Nineteenth-Century America*. Boston: Beacon Press, 1989.

Brett, Matthew. *The MNI Brain and the Talairach Atlas*. MRC Cognition and Brain Sciences Unit, 1999. Available at http://www.mrc-cbu.cam.ac.uk/imaging/mnispace.html. Accessed 2001.

Brodie, J. D., A. P. Wolf, N. Volkow, et al. "Evaluation of Regional Glucose Metabolism with Positron Emission Tomography in Normal and Psychiatric

Populations." In *Positron Emission Tomography of the Brain*, eds., W.-D. Heiss and Michael E. Phelps. Berlin: Springer-Verlag, 1983.

Browner, Carol, and Nancy Press. "Production of Authoritative Knowledge in American Prenatal Care." 10, no. 2 (1996): 141–156.

Brucer, Marshall. "Nuclear Medicine Begins with a Boa Constrictor." *Journal of Nuclear Medicine* 19 (1978): 581–598.

Buchsbaum, M. S., L. E. DeLisi, H. H. Holcomb, et al. "Cerebral Glucography in Schizophrenia." In *Metabolism of the Human Brain Studied with Positron Emission Tomography*. ed., Greitz, T., D. H. Ingvar, and L. Widen, pp. 471*ff*. New York: Raven Press, 1985.

Burke, Kenneth. *A Grammar of Motives*. New York: Prentice Hall, 1945.

———. *Language as Symbolic Action: Essays on Life, Literature, and Method*. Berkeley: University of California Press, 1966.

Buytendijk, F.J.J. *Prolegomena to an Anthropological Physiology*. Duquesne Studies. Psychological Series, vol. 6. Pittsburgh: Duquesne University Press, 1974.

Canguilhem, Georges. *On the Normal and the Pathological*. Translated from the French by Carolyn R. Fawcett, with Robert S. Cohen; introduction by Michel Foucault. Boston: D. Reidel Publishing, 1978.

———. *Ideology and Rationality in the History of the Life Sciences*. Translated by Arthur Goldhammer. Cambridge, Mass.: MIT Press, 1988.

Caplan, Lincoln. *The Insanity Defense and the Trial of John W. Hinckley, Jr.* Boston: D. R. Godine, 1984.

Carrithers, Michael, Steven Collins, and Steven Lukes. *The Category of the Person: Anthropology, Philosophy, History*. New York: Cambridge University Press, 1985.

Carson, Richard E. "Parameter Estimation in Positron Emission Tomography." In *Positron Emission Tomography and Autoradiography: Principles and Applications for the Brain and Heart*, eds., Michael E. Phelps, John C. Mazziotta, and Heinrich R. Schelbert, pp. 347–390. New York: Raven Press, 1986.

Cartwright, Lisa. *Screening the Body: Tracing Medicine's Visual Culture*. Minneapolis: University of Minnesota Press, 1995.

Castoriadis, C. *Crossroads in the Labyrinth*. Cambridge, Mass.: MIT Press, 1984.

Changeux, Jean-Pierre. *Neuronal Man: The Biology of Mind*. New York: Pantheon Books, 1985.

Charlton, B. G. "A Critique of Biological Psychiatry." *Psychological Medicine* 20, no. 1 (1990): 3–6.

Clarke, Edwin, and Kenneth Dewhurst. *An Iillustrated History of Brain Function*. Berkeley: University of California Press, 1972.

Clarke, Edwin, and L. S. Jacyna. *Nineteenth-Century Origins of Neuroscientific Concepts*. Berkeley: University of California Press, 1987.

Cooter, Roger. *The Cultural Meaning of Popular Science: Phrenology and the Organization of Consent in Nineteenth-Century Britain*. New York: Cambridge University Press, 1984.

Council on Scientific Affairs Reports, American Medical Association. "Positron Emission Tomography—A New Approach to Brain Chemistry." *Journal of the American Medical Association* 260, no. 18 (1988): 2704–2710.

Crary, Jonathan , and Sanford Kwinter. *Incorporations*. New York: Zone, 1992.

Crease, R. P. "Biomedicine in the age of Imaging." *Science* 261, no. 5121 (1993): 554*ff*.

Croft, Barbara Y. "Functional Imaging." In *Functional Mapping of Organ Systems and Other Computer Topics: 11th Annual Symposium on the Sharing of Computer Programs and Technology in Nuclear Medicine*. ed., Peter D. Esser. New York: Society of Nuclear Medicine, 1981.

Csordas, Thomas J. "Embodiment as a Paradigm for Anthropology." *Ethos* 18, no. 1 (1990): 5–47.

———. *Embodiment and Experience: The Existential Ground of Culture and Self*. Cambridge Studies in Medical Anthropology; vol. 2. Cambridge: Cambridge University Press, 1994a.

———. *The Sacred Self: A Cultural Phenomenology of Charismatic Healing*. Berkeley: University of California Press, 1994b.

Danziger, Kurt. *Constructing the Subject: Historical Origins of Psychological Research*. Cambridge Studies in the History of Psychology. Cambridge: Cambridge University Press, 1990a.

———. "Generative Metaphor and the History of Psychological Discourse." In *Metaphors in the History of Psychology*. ed., David E. Leary, pp. 331–356. Cambridge: Cambridge University Press, 1990b.

Daston, Lorraine, and Peter Galison. "The Image of Objectivity." *Representations*, vol. 40 (1992): 81–128.

Daubert v. *Merrell Dow Pharmaceuticals, Inc.* 1993. 113 5. Ct. 2786.

de Lauretis, Teresa. *Alice Doesn't: Feminism, Semiotics, Cinema*. Bloomington: Indiana University Press, 1984.

———. *Technologies of Gender: Essays on Theory, Film, and Fiction*. Bloomington: Indiana University Press, 1987.

DeBenedictis, Don J. "Criminal Minds: PET Scans Used to Prove Accused Killers' Brain Abnormalities." *ABA Journal* Jan. (1990): 30.

Deleuze, Gilles. *Cinema 2: The Time-Image*. Minneapolis: University of Minnesota Press, 1989.

Delgado, Jose M. R. *Physical Control of the Mind: Toward a Psychocivilized Society*. New York: Harper & Row, 1969.

Delisi, Lynn E., and Monte S. Buchsbaum. "Positron Emission Tomography (PET) of Regional Cerebral Glucose Use in Psychiatric Patients." In *New Brain Imaging Techniques and Psychopharmacology*. ed., Michael R. Trimble, pp. 49–62. Oxford: Oxford University Press, 1986.

Dening, G. *History's Anthropology: The Death of William Gooch*. New York: University Press of America, 1988.

Descartes, René. *Philosophical Works of Descartes*. London: Cambridge University Press, 1970.

Diehl, D. J., and M. A. Mintun. "Morning versus Midday Differences in Baseline Regional Cerebral Blood Flow in Healthy Volunteers Demonstrated by PET" (abstract). *Journal of Nuclear Medicine* 38, no. 5 (1995): 128.

Diprose, Rosalyn, and Robyn Ferrell. *Cartographies: Poststructuralism and the Mapping of Bodies and Spaces*. North Sydney, NSW, Australia: Allen & Unwin, 1991.

Douglas, Mary. *Purity and Danger: An Analysis of the Concepts of Pollution and Taboo*. London: Ark, 1966.

Douglas, Mary, and David Hull, eds. *How Classification Works: Nelson Goodman among the Social Sciences*. Edinburgh: Edinburgh University Press, 1992.

Douglas, Mary, and Aaron Wildavsky. *Risk and Culture: An Essay on the Selection of Technological and Environmental Dangers*. Berkeley: University of California Press, 1982.

Downey, Gary Lee, and Joseph Dumit, eds. *Cyborgs and Citadels: Anthropological Interventions in Emerging Sciences and Technologies*. Santa Fe: School of American Research Press, 1997a.

Downey, Gary Lee, and Joseph Dumit. "Locating and Intervening: An Introduction." In *Cyborgs and Citadels: Anthropological Interventions in Emerging Sciences and Technologies*. eds., Gary Lee Downey and Joseph Dumit, pp. 5–29. Santa Fe: School of American Research Press, 1997b.

Dumit, Joseph. "Brain–Mind Machines and American Technological Dream Marketing: Towards an Ethnography of Cyborg Envy." In *Cyborg Handbook*. ed., Chris Hables Gray. New York: Routledge, 1995a.

———. "Twenty-First-Century PET: Looking for Mind and Morality through the Eye of Technology." In *Technoscientific Imaginaries: Conversations, Profiles, and Memoirs*. ed., George E. Marcus, vol. 2, pp. 87–128. Chicago: University of Chicago Press, 1995b.

———. "A Digital Image of the Category of the Person: PET Scanning and Objective Self-Fashioning." In *Cyborgs & Citadels: Anthropological Interventions in Emerging Sciences and Technologies*. eds., Gary Lee Downey and Joseph Dumit. Santa Fe: N.M.: School of American Research Press, 1997, pp. 83–102.

———. "PET Scanner." In *Instruments of Science: An Historical Encyclopedia*, ed., Robert Bud; Garland Encyclopedias in the History of Science. New York: Routledge, 1997.

———. "Objective Brains, Prejudicial Images." *Science in Context* 12, no. 1 (1999): 173–201.

———. "Biology Is Wily." A Paper delivered at the 99th annual meeting of the American Anthropological Association, San Francisco, Nov. 15–19, 2000a.

———. "When Explanations Rest: 'Good-enough' Brain Science and the New Sociomedical Disorders." In *Living and Working with the New Biomedical Technologies: Intersections of Inquiry*. ed., Margaret Lock, Allan Young, and Alberto Cambrosio. Cambridge: Cambridge University Press, 2000b.

———. "Playing Truths: Logics of Seeking and the Persistance of the New Age." *Focaal* 37 (2001): 63–76.

Eccles, John C. *Evolution of the Brain: Creation of the Self*. London: Routledge, 1989.

Eco, Umberto. *A Theory of Semiotics*. Bloomington: Indiana University Press, 1979.

Edgerton, Robert B. *The Cloak of Competence*. Rev'd and updated ed. Berkeley: University of California Press, 1993.

Editorial. "Brain's Singular Way with Language." *Science News* 147 (1995): 202.

Ell, S. R. "Radiology and History" [see comments]. *Investigative Radiology* 23, no. 12 (1988): 956–958.

Estroff, Sue E. "Identity, Disability and Schizophrenia: The Problem of Chronicity." In *Knowledge, Power, and Practice: The Anthropolgy of Medicine and Everday Life*, ed., Shirley Lindenbaum and Margaret M. Lock, pp. 247–286. Berkeley: University of California Press, 1993.

Fabrega, Horacio. "An Ethnomedical Perspective of Anglo-American Psychiatry." *American Journal of Psychiatry* 146 (1989): 588–596.

Farquhar, Judith. "Eating Chinese Medicine." Paper delivered at the 91st annual meeting of the American Anthropological Association, San Francisco, Dec. 2–6, 1992.

Faulstich, M. E., and D. C. Sullivan. "Positron Emission Tomography in Neuropsychiatry." *Investigative Radiology* 26, no. 2 (1991): 184–194.

Fausto-Sterling, Anne. *Sexing the Body: Gender Politics and the Construction of Sexuality*. New York: Basic Books, 2000.

Favret-Saada, Jeane. *Deadly Words: Witchcraft in the Bocage*. Translated by Catherine Cullen [orig. 1977]. Cambridge: Cambridge University Press, 1980.

Fazio, F., D. Perani, M. C. Gilardi, et al. "Metabolic Impairment in Human Amnesia: A PET Study of Memory Networks." *Journal of Cerebral Blood Flow and Metabolism* 12, no. 3 (1992): 353–358.

Fischer, Michael M. J. "Eye(I)ing the Sciences and Their Signifiers (Language, Tropes, Autobiographers): InterViewing for a Cultural Studies of Science and Technology." In *Technoscientific Imaginaries: Conversations, Profiles, and Memoirs*, ed., George E. Marcus, vol. 2, pp. 43–83. Chicago: University of Chicago Press, 1995.

Fleck, Ludwig. *Genesis and Development of a Scientific Fact*. Translated by Fred Bradley and Trenn [orig. 1935]; eds., Thaddeus J. Trenn and Robert K. Merton. Chicago: University of Chicago Press, 1979.

Flusser, Vilém. *Toward a Philosophy of Photography*. Göttingen, West Germany: European Photography, 1984.

Fodor, Jerry. "Diary." *London Review of Books*, 21 (19) September 30, 1999.

Fodor, Jerry A. *The Modularity of Mind: An Essay on Faculty Psychology*. Cambridge, Mass.: MIT Press, 1983.

Ford, Ian. "Can Statistics Cause Brain Damage?" (editorial.) *Journal of Cerebral Blood Flow and Metabolism* 3 (1983): 259–262.

Ford, I., J. H. McColl, A. G. McCormack, and S. J. McCrory. "Statistical Issues in the Analysis of Neuroimages." *Journal of Cerebral Blood Flow and Metabolism* 11, no. 2 (1991): A89–A95.

Fortun, Mike. "The Human Genome Project and the Acceleration of Biotechnology." In *Private Science: Biotechnology and the Rise of the Molecular Sciences*. ed., A. Thackray, Philadelphia: University of Pennsylvania Press, 1988, pp. 182–201.

———. "Mediated Speculations in the Genomics Futures Markets." *New Genetics and Society* 20 (2001): 139–156.

Foucault, Michel. *The History of Sexuality: Volume 1: An Introduction*. Translated by Robert Hurley [orig. 1976]. New York: Vintage Books, 1978.

Foucault, Michel, Luther H. Martin, Huck Gutman, and Patrick H. Hutton, eds. *Technologies of the Self: A Seminar with Michel Foucault.* Amherst: University of Massachusetts Press, 1988.

Fox, J. L. "PET Scan Controversy Aired" [news]. *Science* 224, no. 4645 (1984): 143–144.

Fox, P. T., and J. V. Pardo. "Does inter-subject variability in cortical functional organization increase with neural 'distance' from the periphery?" *CIBA Foundation Symposium* 163 (1991): 125–140; discussion 140–144.

Fox, P. T., J. S. Perlmutter, and M. E. Raichle. "A Stereotactic Method of Anatomical Localization for Positron Emission Tomography." *Journal of Computer Assisted Tomography* 9 (1985): 141–153.

Fox, P. T., and M. G. Woldorff. "Integrating Human Brain Maps." *Current Opinion in Neurobiology* 4, no. 2 (1994): 151–156.

Fox, Robin. *The Challenge of Anthropology: Old Encounters and New Excursions.* New Brunswick, N.J.: Transaction, 1994.

Fox, Robin, and Association of Social Anthropologists of the Commonwealth, eds. *Biosocial Anthropology,* ASA Studies, vol. 1. New York: Wiley, 1975.

Frackowiak, Richard S. J. "An Introduction to Positron Tomography and Its Application to Clinical Investigation." In *New Brain Imaging Techniques and Psychopharmacology.* ed., Michael R Trimble, pp. 25–34. Oxford: Oxford University Press, 1986.

Franconi, Cafiero. "Introduction." In *Applications of Physics to Medicine and Biology: Proceedings of the 2nd International Conference on the Applications of Physics to Medicine and Biology, Trieste, Italy, 7–11 November 1983,* p. 1.

Franklin, Jon. *Molecules of the Mind: The Brave New Science of Molecular Psychology.* New York: Atheneum, 1987.

Franklin, Sarah, and Helene Ragone. *Reproducing Reproduction: Kinship, Power, and Technological Innovation.* Philadelphia: University of Pennsylvania Press, 1998.

Friedkin, William, and William P. Wood. *Rampage* (screenplay). From the motion picture produced by De Laurentiis Entertainment Group, 1988. Videocassette distributed by Paramount Home Video, 1992.

Frith, C. "Positron Emission Tomography Studies of Frontal Lobe Function: Relevance to Psychiatric Disease." *CIBA Foundation Symposium* 163 (1991): 181–191; discussion, 191–197.

Froehlich, Cliff. "Mapping the Brain: PET Researchers Establish New Connections between the Mind's Activity and the Brain's Anatomy." *Focal Spot* 18, no. 2 (1987): 14–21.

Frye v. *United States.* 1923. 293 F. 1013, 1014, D.C.Cir.

Gagliardi, R. A. "The Academic Medical Expert Witness. A New Confrontation between Town and Gown." *Investigative Radiology* 23, no. 8 (1988): 636–638.

Galison, Peter Louis. *Image and Logic: A Material Culture of Microphysics.* Chicago: University of Chicago Press, 1997.

Gazzaniga, M. S. "Organization of the Human Brain." *Science* 245, no. 4921 (1989): 947–952.

Geertz, Clifford. "The Growth of Culture and the Evolution of Mind." In *The Interpretation of Cultures.* ed., Clifford Geertz. New York: Basic Books, 1973.

215

Gewertz, Deborah B., and Edward L. Schieffelin. *History and Ethnohistory in Papua New Guinea*. Oceania Monograph, vol. 28. Sydney: University of Sydney, 1985.

Gilman, Sander L. *Disease and Representation: Images of Illness from Madness to AIDS*. Ithaca: Cornell University Press, 1988.

Ginsburg, Faye, and Rayna Rapp. *Conceiving the New World Order*. Berkeley: University of California Press, 1995.

Gjedde, A, and H. Kuwabara. "Absent Recruitment of Capillaries in Brain Tissue Recovering from Stroke." *Acta Neurochirurgica Supplement* 57 (1993): 35–40.

Golan, Tal. "History of Scientific Expert Testimony in Common Law Courts." *Science in Context* 12 (1999): 7–32.

———. "The Authority of Shadows: The Legal Embrace of the X-ray." *Historical Reflections/Réflexions Historiques* 24 (1998): 437–458.

Gombrich, E. H. "Illusion and Art." In *Illusion in Nature and Art*. eds., R. L. Gregory, E. H. Gombrich, and Colin Blakemore. New York: Scribner, 1973, pp. 208–230.

Good, Byron J. *Medicine, Rationality and Experience: An Anthropological Perspective*. Lewis Henry Morgan Lecture Series. Cambridge: Cambridge University Press, 1994.

Good, Mary-Jo, P. Brodwin, Byron J. Good, and Arthur Kleinman, eds. *Pain as Human Experience: An Anthropological Perspective*. Berkeley: University of California Press, 1992.

Good, Mary-Jo Del Vecchio, Tseunetsugu Munakata, Yasuki Kobayashi, et al. "Oncology and Narrative Time." *Social Science Medicine* 38, no. 6 (1994): 855–862.

Goodman, Nelson. *Fact, Fiction, and Forecast*, 3d ed. Indianapolis: Bobbs-Merrill, 1973.

———. "Seven Strictures on Similarity." In *How Classification Works: Nelson Goodman among the Social Sciences*. eds., Mary Douglas and David Hull, pp. 13–23. Edinburgh: Edinburgh University Press, 1992.

Grady, C. L. "Quantitative Comparison of Measurements of Cerebral Glucose Metabolic Rate Made with Two Positron Cameras." *Journal of Cerebral Blood Flow and Metabolism* 11, no. 2 (1991): A57–A63.

Greimas, Algirdas-Julien, and Jacques Fontanille. *The Semiotics of Passions: From States of Affairs to States of Feeling*. Minneapolis: University of Minnesota Press, 1993.

Greimas, A.-J. , and J. Courtes. *Semiotics and Language: An Analytical Dictionary*. Bloomington: Indiana University Press, 1982.

Grosz, Elizabeth A. *Volatile Bodies: Toward a Corporeal Feminism (Theories of Representation and Difference)*. Bloomington: Indiana University Press, 1994.

Guilshan, Christine A. "A Picture Is Worth a Thousand Lies: Electronic Imaging and the Future of the Admissibility of Photographs into Evidence." *Rutgers Computer and Technology Law Journal* 18 (1992): 365–380.

Gur, R. C., R. E. Gur, W. D. Obrist, et al. "Sex and Handedness differences in Cerebral Blood Flow during Rest and Cognitive Activity." *Science* 217, no. 4560 (1982): 659–661.

216

Gur, R. C., L. H. Mozley, P. D. Mozley, et al. "Sex Differences in Regional Cerebral Glucose Metabolism during a Resting State." *Science* 267, no. 5197 (1995): 528–531.

Gur, R. C., J. D. Ragland, S. M. Resnick, et al. "Lateralized Increases in Cerebral Blood Flow during Performance of Verbal and Spatial Tasks: Relationship with Performance Level." *Brain and Cognition* 24, no. 2 (1994): 244–258.

Gur, Ruben C., and Raquel E. Gur. "The Use of Neuroimaging Techniques in Brain Injury." In *Neuropsychology and the Law.* eds., Jane Dywan, Ronald D. Kaplan, and Francis J. Pirozzolo, pp. 164–185. New York: Springer-Verlag, 1991.

Gusterson, Hugh. *Nuclear Rites: A Weapons Laboratory at the End of the Cold War.* Berkeley: University of California Press, 1996.

Hacking, Ian. *Representing and Intervening: Introductory Topics in the Philosophy of Natural Science.* Cambridge: Cambridge University Press, 1983.

Halperin, Edward C. "X-rays at the Bar, 1896–1910." *Investigative Radiology* 22 (1988): 639–646.

Haraway, Donna J. *Simians, Cyborgs, and Women: The Reinvention of Nature.* London: Free Association Books, 1991.

Harding, Susan. "Convicted by the Holy Spirit: The Rhetoric of Fundamental Baptist Conversion." *American Ethnologist* 14, no. 1 (1987): 167–181.

Harding, Sandra. *Whose Science? Whose Knowledge?: Thinking from Women's Lives.* Ithaca, N.Y.: Cornell University Press, 1991.

Harrington, Anne. *Medicine, Mind, and the Double Brain: A Study in Nineteenth-Century Thought.* Princeton, N.J.: Princeton University Press, 1987.

Harrington, Anne, ed. *So Human a Brain: Knowledge and Values in the Neurosciences.* Boston: Dibner Institute Publication/Birkhauser, 1992.

Harris, Juliana. "Illuminating mysteries of the brain." *UCLA Medicine* spring (1990): 15–18.

Harris, Neil. *Humbug: The Art of P. T. Barnum.* Boston: Little, Brown, 1973.

Hartouni, Valerie. "Containing Women: Reproductive Discourse in the 1980s." In *Technoculture.* ed., Constance Penley and Andrew Ross, pp. 27–56. Minneapolis: University of Minnesota Press, 1991.

Hartouni, V. "Fetal Exposures — Abortion Politics and the Optics of Allusion." *Camera Obscura* N29 (1992): 131*ff.*

Hatfield, Scott. "PET May Someday Help Screen for Criminal Behavior, says PhD." *ADVANCE for Radiologic Science Professionals* (1995a) 8: 14.

———. "PET Shows Female Brain Has Evolved More Than Male's." *ADVANCE for Radiologic Science Professionals* (1995b) 8: 14–15.

Hawkins, R. A., and A. L. Miller. "Loss of Radioactive 2-Deoxy-D-Glucose-6-Phosphate from Brains of Conscious Rats: Implications for Quantitative Autoradiographic Determination of Regional Glucose Utilization." *Neuroscience* 3, no. 2 (1978): 251–258.

Heath, Deborah. "Bodies, Antibodies, and Modest Interventions." In *Cyborgs and Citadels: anthropological interventions in emerging sciences and technologies,* ed. Gary Lee Downey and Joseph Dumit. Santa Fe: School of American Research Press, 1997.

Heath, Robin, and Mary Katherine Crabb. "Mind–Body Dualism and the Etiology of Depression." Unpublished manuscript, Department of Anthropology, University of Kentucky, Lexington, 1993.

Heidegger, Martin. *Being and Time*. London: SCM Press, 1962.

Heims, Steve J. *The Cybernetics Group*. Cambridge, Mass.: MIT Press, 1991.

Heiss, W. D., G. Pawlik, V. Holthoff, et al. "PET Correlates of Normal and Impaired Memory Functions." *Cerebrovascular and Brain Metabolism Reviews* 4, no. 1 (1992): 1–27.

Hensler, Timothy B. "Comment: A Critical Look at the Admissability of Polygraph Evidence in the Wake of Daubert: The Lie Detector Fails the Test." *Catholic University Law Review* 46 (1997): 1247.

Hess, David J. *Science and Technology in a Multicultural World: The Cultural Politics of Facts and Artifacts*. New York: Columbia University Press, 1995.

———. *Can Bacteria Cause Cancer?: Alternative Medicine Confronts Big Science*. New York: New York University Press, 1997.

Hixson, Joseph R. "New Seeing-Eye Machines . . . Look Inside Your Body, Can Save Your Life." *Vogue* July (1983): 238–239, 254–258.

Holland, Dorothy C., and Naomi Quinn. *Cultural Models in Language and Thought*. Cambridge: Cambridge University Press, 1987.

Horgan, J. "Fractured Functions. Does the Brain Have a Supreme Integrator?" *Scientific Am* 269, no. 6 (1993): 36–37.

Houts, Marshall. "Presenting the Medical Evidence: Using Brain Scans to Differentiate Stroke from Hypoxia (A Case History Report: $750,000 Verdict)." *Trauma* 27, no. 1 (1985): 11–42.

Huang, M, and R. L. Veech. "The quantitative Determination of the in vivo Dephosphorylation of Glucose 6-Phosphate in Rat Brain." *Journal of Biological Chemistry* 257, no. 19 (1982): 11358–11363.

Huang, Sung-cheng, and Michael E. Phelps. "Principles of Tracer Kinetic Modeling in Positron Emission Tomography and Autoradiography." In *Positron Emission Tomography and Autoradiography: Principles and Applications for the Brain and Heart*. eds., Michael E. Phelps, John C. Mazziotta, and Heinrich R. Schelbert, pp. 287–346. New York: Raven Press, 1986.

Huff, Darrell. *How to Lie with Statistics*. New York: Norton, 1954.

Hull, David. "Biological Species: An Inductivist's Nightmare." In *How Classification Works: Nelson Goodman among the Social Sciences*. eds., Mary Douglas and David Hull, pp. 42–68. Edinburgh: Edinburgh University Press, 1992.

Huntington v. Crowley. 1966. 54 Cal.2d 647.

International Atomic Energy Agency. "Radiopharmaceuticals from Generator-Produced Radionuclides," Proceedings of a panel. Vienna, 1971.

Irigaray, Luce. *Sexes and Genealogies*. New York: Columbia University Press, 1993.

Jackson, Jean. "Chronic Pain and the Tension between the Body as Subject and Object." In *Embodiment and Experience: The Existential Ground of Culture and Self*. ed., Thomas J. Csordas. Cambridge: Cambridge University Press, 1994.

———. *Camp Pain: Talking with Chronic Pain Patients*. Philadelphia: University of Pennsylvania Press, 2000.

James, William. *The Principles of Psychology: American Science — Advanced Course*. New York: H. Holt and Company, 1970 (1890).

Jardine, Nicholas. "The Laboratory Revolution in Medicine as Rhetorical and Aesthetic Accomplishment." In *The Laboratory Revolution in Medicine*. eds., Andrew Cunningham and Perry Williams, pp. 304–323. Cambridge: Cambridge University Press, 1992.

Jasanoff, Sheila. *Science at the Bar: Law, Science, and Technology in America*. Cambridge, Mass: Harvard University Press, 1995.

Jeannerod, Marc. *The Brain Machine: The Development of Neurophysiological Thought*. Cambridge, Mass.: Harvard University Press, 1985.

Jeffery, C. Ray. "The Brain, the Law, and the Medicalization of Crime." In *The Neurotransmitter Revolution: Serotonin, Social Behavior, and the Law*. eds., Roger D. Masters and Michael T. McGuire, pp. 161–178. Carbondale: Southern Illinois University Press, 1994.

Johnson, Thomas M., and Carolyn Fishel Sargent, eds. *Medical Anthropology: A Handbook of Theory and Method*. New York: Greenwood Press, 1990.

Jones, Caroline A., Peter Louis Galison, and Amy E Slaton, eds. *Picturing Science, Producing Art*. New York: Routledge, 1998.

Kaihara, S., T. K. Natarajan, C. D. Maynard, and H. N. Wagner Jr. "Construction of a Functional Image from Spatially Localized Rate Constants Obtained from Serial Camera and Rectilinear Scanner Data." *Radiology* 93 (1969): 1345–1348.

Kant, Immanuel. *Anthropology from a Pragmatic Point of View*. Carbondale, Ill.: Southern Illinois University Press, 1978.

Kant, Immanuel. *Critique of Judgment*. Werner S. Pluhar. Indianapolis: Hackett Publishing, 1987.

Kaplan, Bonnie. "Computers in Medicine." Doctoral dissertation, University of Chicago, 1983.

Karp, J. S., M. E. Daube-Witherspoon, and G. Muehllehner. "Factors Affecting Accuracy and Precision in PET Volume Imaging." *Journal of Cerebral Blood Flow and Metabolism* 11, no. 2 (1991): A38–A44.

Kearfott, K. J., D. A. Rottenberg, and R. J. Knowles. "A New Headholder for PET, CT, and NMR Imaging." *Journal of Computer Assisted Tomography* 8, no. 6 (1984): 1217–1220.

Keesing, Roger. "Colonial History as Contested Ground: The Bell Massacre in the Solomons." *History and Anthropology* 4 (1990): 279–301.

Keller, Evelyn Fox. *A Feeling for the Organism: The Life and Work of Barbara McClintock*. San Francisco: W.H. Freeman, 1983.

Kenny, Lorraine. "Qualifying Essay." Qualifying Essay, University of California at Santa Cruz, 1992.

Kereiakes, J. G. "The History and Development of Medical Physics Instrumentation: Nuclear Medicine." *Medical Physics* 14, no. 1 (1987): 146–155.

Kevles, Bettyann Holtzmann. *Naked to the Bone: Medical Imaging in the Twentieth Century*. New Brunswick, N.J.: Rutgers University Press, 1997.

Kilbourn, M. R., and M. R. Zalutsky. "Research and Clinical Potential of Receptor-Based Radiopharmaceuticals." *Journal of Nuclear Medicine* 26, no. 6 (1985): 655–662.

219

Kingsley, D. P., M. Bergstrom, and B. M. Berggren. "A Critical Evaluation of Two Methods of Head Fixation." *Neuroradiology* 19, no. 1 (1980): 7–12.

Kittler, Friedrich A. *Discourse Networks 1800/1900.* Translated by Michael Metteer and Chris Cullens. Stanford: Stanford University Press, 1985.

Klein, D., B. Milner, R. J. Zatorre, et al. "The Neural Substrates Underlying Word Generation: A Bilingual Functional-Imaging Study." *Proceedings of the National Academy of Sciences of the United States of America* 92, no. 7 (1995): 2899–2903.

Klein, D., R. J. Zatorre, B. Milner, et al. "Left Putaminal Activation When Speaking a Second Language: Evidence from PET." *Neuroreport* 5, no. 17 (1994): 2295–2297.

Kleinman, Arthur, and Byron Good, eds. *Culture and Depression: Studies in the Anthropology and Cross-Cultural Psychiatry of Affect and Disorder.* Comparative Studies of Health Systems and Medical Care, vol. 16. Berkeley: University of California Press, 1985.

Kleinman, A., and J. Kleinman. "Suffering and Its Professional Transformation: Toward an Ethnography of Interpersonal Experience." *Culture, Medicine and Psychiatry* 15, no. 3 (1991): 275–301.

Knight, Nancy. "The New Light: X-Rays and Medical Futurism." In *Imagining Tomorrow: History, Technology and the American Future.* ed., Joseph J. Corn. Cambridge, Mass.: MIT Press, 1986.

Knorr-Cetina, K. *Epistemic Cultures: How the Sciences Make Knowledge.* Cambridge, Mass.: Harvard University Press, 1999.

Koch, Ellen Breckenridge. "The Process of Innovation in Medical Technology: American research on Ultrasound, 1947 to 1962." Doctoral dissertation, University of Pennsylvania, Philadelphia, 1990.

Koeppe, R. A., and G. D. Hutchins. "Instrumentation for Positron Emission Tomography: Tomographs and Data Processing and Display Systems." *Seminars in Nuclear Medicine* 22, no. 3 (1992): 162–181.

Konner, Melvin. *The Tangled Wing: Biological Constraints on the Human Spirit.* New York: Holt, Rinehart, and Winston, 1982.

———. *Medicine at the Crossroads: The Crisis in Health Care.* New York: Pantheon Books, 1993.

Kopytoff, Igor. "The Cultural Biography of Things: Commoditization as Process." In *The Social Life of Things: Commodities in Cultural Perspective.* Arjun Appadurai, ed. pp. 64–93. Cambridge, Cambridge University Press, 1986.

Kosslyn, S. M. "The Psychology of Visual Displays." *Investigative Radiology* 24, no. 5 (1989): 417–419.

———. *Image and Brain: The Resolution of the Imagery Debate.* Cambridge, Mass.: MIT Press, 1994.

Kosslyn, Stephen Michael, and Olivier Koenig. *Wet Mind: The New Cognitive Neuroscience.* New York: Free Press, 1992.

Kramer, Peter D. *Listening to Prozac: A Psychiatrist Explores Antidepressant Drugs and the Remaking of the Self.* New York: Viking, 1993.

Krech III, Shepard. "The State of Ethnohistory." *Annual Review of Anthropology* 20 (1991): 345–375.

Kruger, Lorenz, Lorraine J. Daston, and Michael Heidelberg, eds. *The Probabilistic Revolution. Vol. 1. Ideas in History.* Cambridge, Mass.: MIT Press, 1987a.

Kruger, Lorenz, Gerd Gigerenzer, and Mary S. Morgan, eds. *The Probabilistic Revolution. Vol. 2. Ideas in the Sciences.* Cambridge, Mass.: MIT Press, 1987b.

Kuhar, Michael J. "Perspectives." In *Brain Imaging: Techniques and Applications.* N. A. Sharif and M. E. Lewis, eds., pp. 13–17. New York: Halsted Press, 1989.

———. "Introduction to Neurotransmitters and Neuroreceptors." In *Quantitative Imaging: Neuroreceptors, Neurotransmitters, and Enzymes.* J. James Frost and Henry N. Wagner Jr., eds. New York: Raven Press, 1990.

Kuhl, D. E., E. J. Metter, W. H. Riege, and M. E. Phelps. "Effects of Human Aging on Patterns of Local Cerebral Glucose Utilization Determined by the [18F]Fluorodeoxyglucose Method." *Journal of Cerebral Blood Flow and Metabolism* 2, no. 2 (1982): 163–171.

Kuhn, Thomas S. *The Structure of Scientific Revolutions.* International Encyclopedia of Unified Science. Foundations of the Unity of Science, vol. 2, no. 2. Chicago: University of Chicago Press, 1970.

Kulynych, Jennifer. "Psychiatric Neuroimaging Evidence: A High-Tech Crystal Ball?" *Stanford Law Review* 49, May (1997): 1249–1270.

Kwong, K. K., J. W. Belliveau, D. A. Chesler, et al. "Dynamic Magnetic Resonance Imaging of Human Brain Activity During Primary Sensory Stimulation." *Proceedings of the National Academy of Science of the United States of America* 89, no. 12 (1992): 5675–5679.

Lassen, N. A., D. H. Ingvar, and E. Skinhoj. "Brain Function and Blood Flow." *Scientific American* 239(4): 62–71, 1978.

Latour, Bruno. *Science in Action: How to Follow Scientists and Engineers through Society.* Cambridge, Mass.: Harvard University Press, 1987.

———. *The Pasteurization of France.* Cambridge, Mass: Harvard University Press, 1988.

Latour, Bruno, and Steve Woolgar. *Laboratory Life: The Construction of Scientific Facts.* Princeton, N.J.: Princeton University Press, 1979.

Lelling, Andrew E. "Comment: Eliminative Materialism, Neuroscience, and the Criminal Law." *University of Pennsylvania Law Review* 141, no. April (1993): 1471–1565.

Leo, John. "Sex: It's All in Your Brain." (column). *U.S. News & World Report* 118, no. 8 (1995): 22(1).

LeVay, Simon. *The Sexual Brain.* Cambridge, Mass: MIT Press, 1993.

Levin, D. M., and G. F. Solomon. "The Discursive Formation of the Body in the History of Medicine." *Journal of Medicine and Philosophy* 15, no. 5 (1990): 515–537.

Levine, Geoffrey, and Neil Abel. "Investigational New Drugs: Application, Process, and Trial." *Journal of Nuclear Medicine Technology* 18, no. 4 (1990): 236–244.

Levi-Strauss, Claude. *Totemism.* Translated by Rodney Needham [1962]. Boston: Beacon Press, 1963.

221

Levi-Strauss, Claude. *The Savage Mind*. The Nature of Human Society (series). Chicago: University of Chicago Press, 1966.

Levy, Robert I. "Emotion, Knowing, and Culture." In *Culture Theory: Essays on Mind, Self, and Emotion*. Richard A. Schweder and Robert A. LeVine, eds. pp. 214–237. Cambridge: Cambridge University Press, 1984.

Luria, A. R. *The Working Brain; An Introduction to Neuropsychology*. New York: Basic Books, 1973.

Lutz, Catherine. *Unnatural Emotions: Everyday Sentiments on a Micronesian Atoll and Their Challenge to Western Theory*. Chicago: University of Chicago Press, 1988.

Lynch, Michael. *Scientific Practice and Ordinary Action: Ethnomethodology and Social Studies of Science*. Cambridge: Cambridge University Press, 1993.

Lynch, Michael, and Samuel Y. Edgerton Jr. "Aesthetics and Digital Image Processing: Representational Craft in Contemporary Astronomy." In *Picturing Power: Visual Depiction and Social Relations*. Gordon Fyfe and John E. Law, eds., pp. 184–220. London: Routledge, 1988.

Lynch, Michael, and Steve Woolgar, eds. *Representation in Scientific Practice*. Cambridge, Mass.: MIT Press, 1990.

MacCormac, E. R. "Images: Cultural, Perceptual, and Computational." *Investigative Radiology* 24, no. 4 (1989): 331–333.

Maisey, M. N. "The Quest for an Image of Man: Diagnostic Medical Imaging." *Lancet* no. 2, 1989, 1493–500..

Makela, Klaus, Alcoholics Anonymous, and World Health Organization, Regional Office for Europe. *Alcoholics Anonymous as a Mutual-Help Movement: A Study in Eight Societies*. Madison, Wisc.: University of Wisconsin Press, 1996.

Manning, Peter, and Horatio Fabrega. "The Experience of Self and Body: Health and Illness in the Chiapas Highlands." In *Phenomenological Sociology*, George Psathas, ed., pp. 59–73. New York: Wiley, 1973.

Marcus, George E., ed. *Technoscientific Imaginaries: Conversations, Profiles, and Memoirs*. Ed., George E. Marcus. Vol. 2, *Late Editions: Cultural Studies for the End of the Century*. Chicago: University of Chicago Press, 1995.

Marks, Harry M. *The Progress of Experiment: Science and Therapeutic Reform in the United States, 1900–1990*. Cambridge History of Medicine. New York: Cambridge University Press, 1997.

Martell, Daniel A. "Forensic Neuropsychology and the Criminal Law." *Law and Human Behavior* 16, no. 3 (1992): 313–336.

Martin, Emily. *The Woman in the Body: A Cultural Analysis of Reproduction*. Boston: Beacon Press, 1987.

———. "Science and Women's Bodies: Forms of Anthropological Knowledge." In *Body/Politics: Women and the Discourses of Science*. Evelyn Fox Keller and Sally Shuttleworth Mary Jacobus, eds., pp. 69–82. New York: Routledge, 1990.

———. *Flexible Bodies: Tracking Immunity in American Culture from the Days of Polio to the Age of AIDS*. Boston: Beacon Press, 1994.

Martin, Neil, Scott Grafton, Fernando Vinuela, et al. "Imaging Techniques for

Cortical Functional Localization." *Clinical Neurosurgery: Congress of Neurological Surgeons* 38 (1990).

Masters, Roger D., and Michael T. McGuire, eds. *The Neurotransmitter Revolution: Serotonin, Social Behavior and the Law.* Carbondale, Ill.: Southern Illinois University Press, 1994.

Mattingly, Cheryl. "The Concept of Therapeutic 'Emplotment'." *Social Science and Medicine* 38, no. 6 (1994): 811–822.

Mauss, Marcel. "A Category of the Human Mind: The Notion of Person; the Notion of Self." In *The Category of the Person.* Michael Carrithers, Steven Collins, and Steven Lukes, eds., pp. 1–25. Cambridge: Cambridge University Press, 1985.

Mayberg, Helen S. "Functional Brain Scans as Evidence in Criminal Court: An Argument for Caution." *Journal of Nuclear Medicine* 33, no. 6 (1992): 18 *ff*.

Mazziotta, J. C. "Physiologic Neuroanatomy: New Brain Imaging Methods Present a Challenge to an Old Discipline." *Journal of Cerebral Blood Flow and Metabolism* 4, no. 4 (1984): 481–483.

Mazziotta, J. C., M. E. Phelps, A. K. Meadors, et al. "Anatomical Localization Schemes for Use in Positron Computed Tomography Using a Specially Designed Headholder." *Journal of Computer Assisted Tomography* 6, no. 4 (1982): 848–853.

Mazziotta, J. C., M. E. Phelps, D. Plummer, and D. E. Kuhl. "Quantitation in Positron Emission Computed Tomography: 5. Physical — Anatomical Effects." *Journal of Computer Assisted Tomography* 5, no. 5 (1981): 734–743.

Mazziotta, J. C., A. W. Toga, A. Evans, et al. "A Probabilistic Atlas of the Human Brain: Theory and Rationale for Its Development. The International Consortium for Brain Mapping (ICBM)." *NeuroImage* 2, no. 2 (1995): 89–101.

Mazziotta, J. C., D. Valentino, S. Grafton, et al. "Relating Structure to Function in vivo with Tomographic Imaging." *CIBA Foundation Symposium* 163 (1991): 93–101; discussion, 101–112.

Mazziotta, J. C., and S. H. Koslow. "Assessment of Goals and Obstacles in Data Acquisition and Analysis from Emission Tomography: Report of a Series of International Workshops." *Journal of Cerebral Blood Flow and Metabolism* 7 (1987): S1–S31.

Mazziotta, J. C., and M. E. Phelps. "Human Neuropsychological Imaging Studies of Local Brain Metabolism: Strategies and Results." *Research Publications — Association for Research in Nervous and Mental Disease* 63 (1985): 121–137.

McCann, U. D., Z. Szabo, U. Scheffel, et al. "Positron Emission Tomographic Evidence of Toxic Effect of MDMA ('Ecstasy') on Brain Serotonin Neurons in Human Beings." *Lancet* 352, no. 9138 (1998): 1433–1437.

McCloud, Scott. *Understanding Comics: The Invisible Art.* Northampton, Mass.: Kitchen Sink Press, 1993.

Menzies, R. J., C. D. Webster, and D. S. Sepejak. "The Dimensions of Dangerousness: Evaluating the Accuracy of Psychometric Predictions of Violence among Forensic Patients." *Law and Human Behavior* 9 (1985): 35–56.

Merleau-Ponty, Maurice. *Signs*. Translated by Richard C. McCleary. Evanston, Ill.: Northwestern University Press, 1964.

Mestrovic, Stjepan G., and John A. Cook. "The Dangerous Standard: What Is It and How Is It Used?" *International Journal of Law and Psychiatry* 8 (1986): 443–469.

Metter, E. J. "Brain-Behavior Relationships in Aphasia Studied by Positron Emission Tomography." *Annals of the New York Academy of Sciences* 620 (1991): 153–164.

Metz, John. "Psychiatric Diagnosis with PET More Difficult Than Expected." *Diagnostic Imaging* (1989) 14: 121–126.

Meyer, A. "The Frontal Lobe Syndrome, the Aphasias and Related Conditions. A Contribution to the History of Cortical Localization." *Brain* 97 (1974): 565–600.

Michael, Robert T. *Sex in America: A Definitive Survey*. Boston: Little, Brown, 1994.

Mintun, M. A., P. T. Fox, and E. M. Raichle. "A Highly Accurate Method of Localizing Regions of Neuronal Activation in the Human Brain with Positron Emission Tomography." *Journal of Cerebral Blood Flow Metabolism* 9, no. 1 (1989): 96–103.

Mitchell, Lisa M., and Eugenia Georges. "Baby's First Picture: The Cyborg Fetus of Ultrasound Imaging." In *Cyborg Babies: From Techno-Sex to Techno-Tots*, Robbie Davis-Floyd and Joseph Dumit, eds., pp. 105–124. New York: Routledge, 1998.

Mnookin, Jennifer. "The Image of Truth: Photographic Evidence and the Power of Analogy." *Yale Journal of Law & the Humanities* 10 (1998): 1.

Monahan, John. "Risk Assessment of Violence among the Mentally Disordered: Generating Useful Knowledge." *International Journal of Law and Psychiatry* 11 (1988): 249–257.

Monahan, John, and Saleem A. Shah. "Dangerousness and Committment of the Mentally Disordered in the United States." *Schizophrenia Bulletin* 15, no. 4 (1989): 541–553.

Montgomery, Geoffrey. "The Mind in Motion (Neurologists Try to Unlock the Secrets of Language)." *Discover* (1989), 10:58(8).

Morse, Stephen J. "Treating Crazy People Less Specially." *West Virginia Law Review* 90 (1988): 353.

Mulvey, E. P., and C. W. Lidz. "Clinical Considerations in the Prediction of Dangerousness in Mental Patients." *Clinical Psychology Review* 4 (1984): 379–401.

Murphy, Brian. "Color Scales: Dialing a Defect." 1996. Available at http://www.nucmed.buffalo.edu/nrlgy1.htm. Accessed March 4, 2003.

Myers, Greg. *Writing Biology: Texts in the Social Construction of Scientific Knowledge*. Madison, Wisc: University of Wisconsin Press, 1990.

National Commission on the Insanity Defense (U.S.) and National Mental Health Association (U.S.). *Myths & Realities: Hearing Transcript of the National Commission on the Insanity Defense*. Arlington, Va., 1983.

Nelkin, Dorothy. *Controversy, Politics of Technical Decisions*. Beverly Hills, Calif.: Sage Publications, 1979.

————. *Selling Science: How the Press Covers Science and Technology*. New York: W. H. Freeman, 1987.

Nelkin, Dorothy, and Laurence Tancredi. *Dangerous Diagnostics: The Social Power of Biological Information*. New York: Basic Books, 1989.

Nelson, T., G. Lucignani, S. Atlas, et al. "Reexamination of Glucose-6-Phosphatase Activity in the Brain in vivo: No Evidence for a Futile Cycle." *Science* 229, no. 4708 (1985): 60–62.

Nice, C. M., Jr. "Medical Images: Past, Present, and Future." *Critical Reviews in Diagnostic Imaging* 14, no. 1 (1980): 73–109.

National Institutes of Health. *The Human Brain Project: Phase I Feasability Studies*. Vol. PA-93-068 Program Annoucement. Bethesda, Md., 1993.

Office of Technology Assessment. *The Biology of Mental Disorders: New Developments in Neuroscience*. U.S. Government Printing Office, 1992, OTA-BA-538. Available at http://www.wws.princeton.edu/cgi-bin/byteserv.prl/~ota/disk1/1992/9237/923701.pdf.

Ojemann, G. "Individual Variability in Cortical Localizaiton of Language." *Journal of Neurosurgery* 50 (1979): 164–169.

Ojemann, G., J. Ojemann, E. Lettich, and M. Berger. "Coritcal Language Localization in Left, Dominant Hemisphere: An Electrical Stimulation Mapping Investigation in 117 Patients." *Journal of Neurosurgery* 71 (1989): 316–326.

Oldendorf, William H. *The Quest for an Image of Brain: Computerized Tomography in the Perspective of Past and Future Imaging Methods*. New York: Raven Press, 1980.

Pardes, Herbert, and Harold Alan Pincus. "Neuroscience and Psychiatry: An Overview." In *The Integration of Neuroscience and Psychiatry*. Herbert Pardes and Harold Alan Pincus, eds., pp. 1–20. Washington, D.C.: American Psychiatric Press, 1985.

Pasveer, B. "Knowledge of Shadows — The Introduction of X-Ray Images in Medicine." *Sociology of Health and Illness* 11, no. 4 (1989): 361–381.

Pawlik, G. "Positron Emission Tomography and Multiregional Statistical Analysis of Brain Function: From Exploratory Methods for Single Cases to Inferential Tests for Multiple Group Designs." In *Progress in Computer-Assisted Function Analysis*. J. L. Willems, J. H. van Bemmel, and J. Michel, eds., pp. 401–408. Amsterdam: North-Holland, 1988.

Pawlik, G. "Statistical Analysis of Functional Neuroimaging Data: Exploratory versus Inferential Methods." *Journal of Cerebral Blood Flow and Metabolism* 11, no. 2 (1991): A136-A139.

Pawlik, G., and W.-D. Heiss. "Positron Emission Tomography and Neuropsychological Function." In *Neuropsychological Function and Brain Imaging*, eds., Erin D. Bigler, Eric Turkheimer, and Ronald A. Yeo. New York: Plenum, 1989.

Pêcheux, Michel. *Language, Semantics, and Ideology: Stating the Obvious. Language, Discourse, Society*. London: Macmillan Press, 1982.

Pechura, Constance M., and Joseph B. Martin. *Mapping the Brain and its Functions: Integrating Enabling Technologies into Neuroscience Research*. Washington, D.C.: National Academy Press, 1991.

People v. Gray. 1986. 187 Cal.App.3d 220. Cal.App.2 Dist.

225

People v. *Kelly*. 1976. 17 Cal.3d 24.

People v. *MacDonald* 1984. 37 Cal. 3d 351.

People v. *Weinstein*. 1992. 591 N.Y.S.2d 715.

Perani, D., M. C. Gilardi, S. F. Cappa, and F. Fazio. "PET Studies of Cognitive Functions: A Review." *Journal of Nuclear Biology and Medicine* 36, no. 4 (1992): 324–336.

Perlin, Michael L. "Unpacking the Myths: The Symbolism Mythology of Insanity Defense Jurisprudence." *Case Western Law Review* 40 (1990): 599.

Perlmutter, J. S., and M. E. Raichle. "In vitro or in vivo Receptor Binding: Where Does the Truth Lie?" [editorial]. *Annals of Neurology* 19, no. 4 (1986): 384–385.

Petersen, Steven E., Peter T. Fox, Michael I. Posner, et al. "Postron Emission Tomographic Studies of the Processing of Single Words." *Journal of Cognitive Neuroscience* 1, no. 2 (1989): 153–170.

Phelps, M. E., and J. C. Mazziotta. "Positron Emission Tomography: Human Brain Function and Biochemistry." *Science* 228, no. 4701 (1985): 799–809.

Phelps, Michael E. "The Evolution of Positron Emission Tomography." In *The Enchanted Loom: Chapters in the History of Neuroscience*, Pietro Corsi, ed., pp. 347–357. New York: Oxford University Press, 1991.

———. "Positron Computed Tomography Studies of Cerebral Glucose Metabolism in Man: Theory and Application in Nuclear Medicine." *Seminars in Nuclear Medicine* 11, no. 1 (1981): 32–49.

Phelps, M. E., E. J. Hoffman, N. A. Mullani, and M. M. Ter-Pogossian. "Application of Annihilation Coincidence Detection to Transaxial Reconstruction Tomography." *Journal of Nuclear Medicine* 16, no. 3 (1975): 210–224.

Poeppel, David. "A Critical Review of PET Studies of Phonological Processing." *Brain and Language* 55 (1996): 317–351.

Pollock, Nathan L. "Accounting for Predictions of Dangerous." *International Journal of Law and Psychiatry* 13 (1990): 207–215.

Poovey, Mary. *A History of the Modern Fact: Problems of Knowledge in the sciences of wealth and society*. Chicago: University of Chicago Press, 1998.

Porter, Theodore. *Trust in Numbers: The Pursuit of Objectivity in Science and Public Life*. Princeton, N.J.: Princeton University Press, 1995.

———. "Quantification and the Accounting Ideal in Science." *Social Studies of Science* 22, no. 4 (1992): 633–652.

Posner, Michael I., and Marcus E. Raichle. *Images of Mind*. New York: Scientific American Library, 1994.

Post, Robert M., and James C. Ballenger, eds. *Neurobiology of Mood Disorders*. Baltimore: Williams & Wilkins, 1984.

Powers, W. J., and M. E. Raichle. "PET: The New Focus of Nuclear Medicine?" letter. *Journal of Nuclear Medicine* 26, no. 12 (1985): 1499–1501.

Prelli, Lawrence J. *A Rhetoric of Science: Inventing Scientific Discourse*. Columbia: University of South Carolina Press, 1989.

Premuda, Loris. "The Historical Development of Neurology: A General Outline." In *PET and NMR: New Perspectives in Neuroimaging and in Clinical Neurochemistry: Proceedings of a Symposium Held in Padova, Italy, May*

15–17, 1985. Leontino Battistin and F. Gerstenbrand, eds., pp. 1–9. New York: A. R. Liss, 1986.

Price, Richard. *First-time: The Historical Vision of an Afro-American People.* Johns Hopkins Studies in Atlantic History and Culture. Baltimore: Johns Hopkins University Press, 1983.

Proctor, Robert. *Value-Free Science? Purity and Power in Modern Knowledge.* Cambridge, Mass.: Harvard University Press, 1991.

Rabinow, Paul. "Artificiality and Enlightenment: From Sociobiology to Bio-sociality." In *Incorporations,* Jonathan Crary and Sanford Kwinter, eds., pp. 190–201. New York: Zone Press, 1992.

Raichle, Marcus E. "Positron Emission Tomography. Progress in Brain Imaging" [news]. *Nature* 317, no. 6038 (1985): 574–576.

————. "Anatomical Explorations of Mind: Studies with Modern Imaging Techniques." *Cold Spring Harbor Symposia on Quantitative Biology* 55 (1990): 983–986.

————. "Images of the Mind: Studies with Modern Imaging Techniques." *Annual Review of Psychology* 45 (1994a): 333–356.

————. "Visualizing the Mind (Brain Imaging)." *Scientific American* (1994b) 58(7).

Rajchman, John. *Michel Foucault: The Freedom of Philosophy.* New York: Columbia University Press, 1985.

Randt, C. T., E. R. Brown, D. P. Osborne Jr. *Randt Memory Test.* New York: New York University, Department of Neurology, 1980.

Rapoport, S. I. "Discussion of PET Workshop Reports, Including Recommendations of PET Data Analysis Working Group." *Journal of Cerebral Blood Flow and Metabolism* 11, no. 2 (1991): A140–A146.

Rapp, Rayna. "Real Time Fetus: The Role of the Sonogram in the Age of Monitored Reproduction." In *Cyborgs and Citadels: Anthropological Interventions in Emerging Sciences and Technologies,* Gary Lee Downey and Joseph Dumit, eds., Santa Fe: School of American Research Press, 1998.

————. *Testing Women, Testing the Fetus: The Social Impact of Amniocentesis in America (The Anthropology of Everyday Life).* New York: Routledge, 1999.

Reiman, E. M. "The Quest to Establish the Neural Substrates of Anxiety." *Psychiatric Clinics of North America* 11, no. 2 (1988): 295–307.

Reiman, Eric M., Maureen J. Fusselman, Peter T. Fox, and Marcus E. Raichle. "Neuroanatomical Correlates of Anticipatory Anxiety." *Science* (1989) 234: 1071(4).

Rein, Harry. "Thermography: Medical and Legal Implications." In *Legal Medicine.* (1986) 4: 95–123.

Reiser, Stanley Joel. *Medicine and the Reign of Technology.* Cambridge: Cambridge University Press, 1978.

Reiser, Stanley Joel, and Michael Anbar, eds. *The Machine at the Bedside: Strategies for Using Technology in Patient Care.* Cambridge: Cambridge University Press, 1984.

Reisner, Ralph, Christopher Slobogin, and Arti Rai. *Law and the Mental Health*

System: Civil and Criminal Aspects, 3d ed. American Casebook Series. St. Paul, Minn.: West Group, 1999.

Reivich, Martin, and Abass Alavi, eds. *Positron Emission Tomography*. New York: Alan R. Liss, 1985.

Reznek, Lawrie. *Evil or Ill?* New York: Routledge, 1997.

Rhodes, Lorna Amarasignham. "Studying Biomedicine as a Cultural System." In *Medical Anthropology: Contemporary Theory and Method*. Thomas M. Johnson and Carolyn F. Sargent, eds., pp. 159–173. New York: Praeger, 1990.

Roberts, L. "Comment: A Call to Action on a Human Brain Project." *Science* 254, no. 5030 (1991): 360.

Robins, L. N. "Psychiatric Epidemiology — A Historic Review." *Social Psychiatry and Psychiatric Epidemiology* 25, no. 1 (1990): 16–26.

Rojas-Burke, J. "PET Scans Advance as Tool in Insanity Defense." *Journal of Nuclear Medicine* 34, no. 1 (1993): N13*ff*.

Roland, Per E. *Brain Activation*. New York: Wiley-Liss, 1993.

Romanucci-Ross, Lola, Daniel E. Moerman, and Laurence R. Tancredi. *The Anthropology of Medicine: From Culture to Method*. New York: Bergin & Garvey, 1991.

Ronell, Avital. *The Telephone Book: Technology — Schizophrenia — Electric Speech*. Lincoln: University of Nebraska Press, 1989.

Rosaldo, Michelle. *Knowledge and Passion: Ilongot Notions of Self and Social Life*. Cambridge: Cambridge University Press, 1980.

———. "Toward an Anthropology of Self and Feeling." In *Culture Theory: Essays on Mind, Self, and Emotion*. Richard Schweder and Robert LeVine eds., pp. 137–157. Cambridge: Cambridge University Press, 1984.

Rose, Nikolas. "The Biology of Culpability: Pathological Identity and Crime Control in a Biological Culture." *Theoretical Criminology* 4, no. 1 (2000): 5–34.

Rose, S., L. L. Kamin, and R. C. Lewontin, eds. *Not in Our Genes: Biology, Ideology, and Human Nature*. Harmondsworth: Penguin, 1984.

Rosser, Sue Vilhauer. *Women's Health — Missing from U.S. Medicine (Race, Gender, and Science)*. Bloomington: Indiana University Press, 1994.

Sacks, W., S. Sacks, and A. Fleischer. "A Comparison of the Cerebral Uptake and Metabolism of Labeled Glucose and Deoxyglucose in vivo in Rats." *Neurochemical Research* 8, no. 5 (1983): 661–685.

Safire, William. "On Language; Only the Factoids." *New York Times Magazine*, 5 December 1993, 32.

Saha, Gobal B., William J. MacIntyre, and Raymundo T. Go. "Cyclotrons and Positron Emission Tomography Radiopharmaceuticals for Clinical Imaging." *Seminars in Nuclear Medicine* 22, no. 3 (1992): 150–161.

Sakurai, Y., T. Momose, M. Iwata, et al. "Kanji Word Reading Process Analysed by Positron Emission Tomography." *Neuroreport* 3, no. 5 (1992): 445–448.

Saunders, Barry Ferguson. "Insection and Decryption: Edgar Poe's 'The Gold Bug' and the Diagnostic Gaze." Master's thesis, University of North Carolina, Chapel Hill, 1989.

Schreiber, Melvyn H. "Ugly Organs." *Investigative Radiology* (1991) 26: 771.

Schulthess, Gustav Konrad von. *Clinical Positron Emission Tomography (PET):*

Correlation with Morphological Cross-Sectional Imaging. Philadelphia: Lippincott, Williams & Wilkins, 2000.

Schwartz, Jeffrey M. *Brain Lock: Free Yourself from Obsessive-Compulsive Behavior: A Four-Step Self-Treatment Method to Change Your Brain Chemistry.* New York: HarperCollins, 1997.

Schweder, Richard A., and Edmund J. Bourne. "Does the Concept of the Person Vary Cross-Culturally?" In *Culture Theory: Essays on Mind, Self, and Emotion.* Richard A. Schweder and Robert A. LeVine, eds., pp. 158–199. Cambridge: Cambridge University Press, 1984.

Schweder, Richard A., and Robert A. LeVine, eds. *Culture Theory: Essays on Mind, Self, and Emotion.* Cambridge: Cambridge University Press, 1984.

Seitz, R. J., and P. E. Roland. "Variability of the Regional Cerebral Blood Flow Pattern Studied with [11C]-Fluoromethane and Position Emission Tomography (PET)." *Computerized Medical Imaging and Graphics* 16, no. 5 (1992): 311–322.

Selbak, John. "Digital Litigation: The Prejudicial Effects of High Technology Animation in the Courtroom." *High Technology Law Journal* 9, no. 2 (1994): 337–367.

Seltzer, Steven E. "Comment on Radiology and History." *Investigative Radiology* 23, no. 12 (1988): 958.

Shannon, Claude E., and Warren Weaver. *The Mathematical Theory of Communication.* Urbana: University of Illinois Press, 1962.

Shapin, S., and S. Schaffer. *Leviathan and the Air-Pump: Hobbes, Boyle, and the Experimental Life.* Princeton, N.J.: Princeton University Press, 1985.

Sheard, M. H. "Clinical Pharmacology of Aggressive Behavior." *Clinical Neuropharmacology* 7 (1984): 173–183.

Shelton, R. C., and D. R. Weinberger. "X-ray Computerized Tomography Studies in Schizophrenia: A Review and Synthesis." In *Handbook of Schizophrenia,* Vol. I: *The Neurology of Schizophrenia.* H. A. Nasrallah and D. R. Weinberger, eds., pp. 207. New York: Elsevier Science, 1986.

Shenton, Martha E., Cynthia G. Wible, and Robert W. McCarley. "A Review of Magnetic Resonance Imaging Studies of Brain Abnormalities in Schizophrenia." In *Brain Imaging in Clinical Psychiatry.* K. Ranga Rama Krishna and P. Murali Doraiswamy, eds., pp. 297–380. New York: Marcel Dekker, 1997.

Shohat, E. "Lasers-For-Ladies—Endo Discourse And the Inscriptions of Science (The Realization of Endometriosis as a Real Disease)." *Camera Obscura* N29 (1992): 57*ff.*

Siegel, Barry A. "Radiopharmaceuticals and FDA: A Clinician's Perspective." *Medical Instrumentation* 15 (1981): 355–360.

Smith, Dorothy E. *Texts, Facts, and Femininity: Exploring the Relations of Ruling.* London: Routledge, 1990.

Smith, Michael R., and Jonathan Brodie. "Positron Emission Tomographic Studies in Schizophrenia: A Review." In *New Brain Imaging Techniques and Psychopharmacology.* Michael R Trimble, ed., pp. 35–48. Oxford: Oxford University Press, 1986.

Smith, Roger. *Inhibition: History and Meaning in the Sciences of Mind and Brain*. Berkeley: University of California Press, 1992.

Sokoloff, Louis. "Basic Principles in the Imaging of Rates of Biochemical Processes in vivo." In *Biomedical Imaging*. Osamu Hayaishi and Kanji Torizuka, eds., p. 183. Tokyo: Academic Press, 1986.

Sokoloff, L., M. Reivich, C. Kennedy, et al. "The [14C]Deoxyglucose Method for the Measurement of Local Cerebral Glucose Utilization: Theory, Procedure, and Normal Values in the Conscious and Anesthetized Albino Rat." *Journal of Neurochemistry* 28 (1977): 897–916.

Solomon, Robert C. "Getting Angry: The Jamesian Theory of Emotion in Anthropology." In *Culture Theory: Essays on Mind, Self, and Emotion*. Richard A. Schweder and Robert A. LeVine, eds., pp. 238–254. Cambridge: Cambridge University Press, 1984.

Spitzer, R. L., J. Endicott, and E. Robins. "Research Diagnostic Criteria." *Psychology and Pharmacology* 11: 22, 1975.

Stafford, Barbara Maria. *Body Criticism: Imaging the Unseen in Enlightenment Art and Medicine*. Cambridge, Mass.: MIT Press, 1991.

Star, Susan Leigh. *Regions of the Mind: Brain Research and the Quest for Scientific Certainty*. Stanford, Calif.: Stanford University Press, 1989.

Star, Susan Leigh. "The Skin, the Skull, and the Self: Toward a Sociology of the Brain." In *So Human a Brain: Knowledge and Values in the Neurosciences*. Anne Harrington, ed., Boston: Birkhauser, 1992.

Starobinski, J. "A Short History of Bodily Sensation." *Psychological Medicine* 20, no. 1 (1990): 23–33.

Starr, Paul. "Social Categories and Claims in the Liberal State." In *How Classification Works: Nelson Goodman among the Social Sciences*. Mary Douglas and David Hull, eds., pp. 154–179. Edinburgh: Edinburgh University Press, 1992.

Stipp, David. "The Insanity Defense in Violent-Crime Cases Gets High-Tech Help." *Wall Street Journal* March 4 (1992): A1*ff.*

Stone, Allucquere Rosanne. "Virtual Systems." In *Incorporations*. Jonathan Crary and Sanford Kwinter, eds., pp. 608–625. New York: Zone Press, 1992.

Storr, Anthony. *Human Aggression*. New York: Bantam Books, 1970.

Stover, G. H. "Medical-Legal Value of the X-ray." *Philadelphia Medical Journal* 2 (1898): 801–802.

Strathern, Marilyn. *Partial Connections*. ASAO special publications; no. 3. Savage, Md.: Rowman & Littlefield Publishers, 1991.

———. *After Nature: English Kinship in the Late Twentieth Century*. The Lewis Henry Morgan Lectures. Cambridge: Cambridge University Press, 1992.

Strother, S. C., J. S. Liow, J. R. Moeller, et al. "Absolute Quantitation in Neurological PET: Do We Need It?" *Journal of Cerebral Blood Flow and Metabolism* 11, no. 2 (1991): A3–A16.

Subramanian, G. "The Role of the Radiochemist in Nuclear Medicine." *Seminars in Nuclear Medicine* 4, no. 3 (1974): 219–227.

Sunder Rajan, Kaushik. "Biocapital: The Constitution of Post-Genomic Life." Dissertation, MIT, Cambridge, Mass., 2002.

Szasz, Thomas Stephen. *Insanity: The Idea and Its Consequences*. New York: Wiley, 1987.

———. *The Meaning of Mind: Language, Morality, and Neuroscience*. Westport, Conn.: Praeger, 1996.

Talairach, J. *Atlas d'anatomie stereotaxique; reperage radiologique indirect des noyaux gris centraux des regions mesencephalo-sous-optique et hypothalamique de l'homme*. Paris: Masson, 1957.

Talairach, J., and Pierre Tournoux. *Co-planar Stereotaxic Atlas of the Human Brain: A 3-Dimensional Proportional System, an Approach to Cerebral Imaging*. Stuttgart: G. Thieme Medical Publishers, 1988.

Taussig, Michael. *The Nervous System*. New York: Routledge, 1991.

———. *Mimesis and Alterity: A Particular History of the Senses*. New York: Routledge, 1993.

Taylor, Janelle S. "Image of Contradiction: Obstetrical Ultrasound in American culture." In *Reproducing Reproduction: Kinship, Power, and Technological Innovation*. Sarah Franklin and Helene Ragone, eds., pp. 15–45. Philadelphia: University of Pennsylvania Press, 1998.

Ter-Pogossian, M. M. "Special Characteristics and Potential for Dynamic Function Studies with PET." *Seminars in Nuclear Medicine* 11, no. 1 (1981): 13–23.

———. "The Origins of Positron Emission Tomography." *Seminars in Nuclear Medicine* 22, no. 3 (1992): 140–149.

Terry, Jennifer. "The Body Invaded: Medical Surveillance of Women as Reproducers." *Socialist Review* 19, July–September (1989): 13–31.

Thompson, Paul Richard. *The Voice of the Past: Oral History* 2nd ed. Oxford: Oxford University Press, 1988.

Thompson, Tracy. *The Beast: A Reckoning with Depression*. New York: G. P. Putnam's Sons, 1995.

Tizard, B. "Theories of Brain Localization from Flourens to Lashley." *Medical History* 3 (1959): 132–145.

Tomkins, J. "'Indians': Textualism, Morality, and the Problem of History." In *"Race," Writing and Difference*. Henry L. Gates, ed., pp. 59–77. Chicago: University of Chicago Press, 1986.

Torrey, E. Fuller. *Surviving Schizophrenia: A Family Manual*. New York: Harper & Row, 1983.

Travers, Bridget, and Jeffrey Muhr. *World of Invention*. Detroit: Gale Research, 1994.

Traweek, Sharon. *Beamtimes and Lifetimes: The World of High Energy Physicists*. Cambridge, Mass.: Harvard University Press, 1988.

Treichler, Paula A. "How to have Theory in an Epidemic: The Evolution of AIDS Treatment Activism." In *Technoculture*. Constance Penley and Andrew Ross, eds., pp. 57–106. Minneapolis: University of Minnesota Press, 1991.

———. *How to Have Theory in an Epidemic: Cultural Chronicles of AIDS*. Durham N.Car.: Duke University Press, 1999.

Turkle, Sherry. *The Second Self: Computers and the Human Spirit*. New York: Simon & Schuster, 1984.

Turner, Victor. "Body, Brain, and Culture." *Zygon* 18, no. 3 (1983): 221–245.

Tyler, Stephen A. *The Unspeakable: Discourse, Dialogue, and Rhetoric in the Postmodern World (Rhetoric of Human Sciences)*. Madison: University of Wisconsin Press, 1987.

Uttal, William R. *The New Phrenology: The Limits of Localizing Cognitive Processes in the Brain (Life and mind)*. Cambridge, Mass.: MIT Press, 2001.

Valentino, Daniel John. "Mapping Human Bbrain Structure–Function Relationships." Dissertation, University of California, Los Angeles, 1991.

Vanier, M., A. R. Lecours, R. Ethier, et al. "Proportional Localization System for Anatomical Interpretation of Cerebral Computed Tomograms." *Journal of Computer Assisted Tomography* 9, no. 4 (1985): 715–724.

Vanoverschelde, Jean-Louis J., William Wijns, Bahija Essamri, et al. "Hemodynamic and Mechanical Determinants of Myocardial O_2 Consumption in Normal Human Heart: Effects of Dobutamine." *American Journal of Physiology* (1993): H1884(9).

Volkow, N. D., J. Brodie, and B. Bendriem. "Positron Emission Tomography: Basic Principles and Applications in Psychiatric Research." *Annals of the New York Academy of Sciences* 620 (1991): 128–144.

Volkow, Nora D., and Alfred P. Wolf, eds. *Positron-Emission Tomography in Schizophrenia Research*. Progress in Psychiatry, no. 33. Washington, D.C.: American Psychiatric Press, 1991.

Wagner, Henry N. "Color in Nuclear Medicine: Contribution or Camouflage?" *Hospital Practice* 9, no. 4 (1974): 87–91.

Wagner, Jr., Henry N. "PET: The New Focus of Nuclear Medicine? Reply." *Journal of Nuclear Medicine* 26, no. 12 (1985): 1500–1501.

———. "Positron Emission Tomography and *In vivo* Brain Chemistry." In *Visualisation of Brain Functions*. eds., D. Ottoson and W. Rostene, vol. 53. New York: Stockton Press, 1989.

Wagner, Jr., Henry N., Robert F. Dannals, James J. Frost, et al. "Imaging Dopamine and Opiate Receptors in the Human Brain in Health and Disease." In *Biomedical Imaging*. ed., Osamu Hayaishi and Kanji Toizuka, pp. 285–296. Tokyo: Academic Press, 1986.

Wagner, Jr., Henry N., and Linda E. Ketchum. *Living with Radiation: The Risk, the Promise*. Baltimore: Johns Hopkins University Press, 1989.

Welch, Michael J., and Michaele R. Gold. *Positron Emission Tomography: The Imaging of Function Rather than Form*, vol. DE-FG02-89 ER 60763. U.S. Department of Energy and Mallinckrodt Institute of Radiology, 1989.

Welch, Michael J., and Michael R. Kilbourn. "Positron Emitters for Imaging." In *Freeman and Johnson's Clinical Radionuclide Imaging*. Leonard M. Freeman and Philip M. Johnson, eds., pp. 181–202. Orlando, Fla.: Grune & Stratton, 1984.

Whitehead, Alfred North. *Modes of Thought*. New York: Macmillan, 1938.

Wiener, Norbert. *Cybernetics; or, Control and Communication in the Animal and the Machine*. Cambridge, Mass.: Hermann Technology Press, 1948.

———. *Cybernetics; or, Control and Communication in the Animal and the Machine*, 2d ed. New York: MIT Press, 1961.

Wiener, Norbert, and J. P. Schade. *Cybernetics of the Nervous System*. Progress in Brain Research, vol. 17. Amsterdam: Elsevier, 1965.

Wilson, Elizabeth A. *Neural Geographies: Feminism and the Microstructure of Cognition.* New York: Routledge, 1998.

Wilson, R. J. "Collimator Technology and Advancements." *Journal of Nuclear Medicine Technology* 1 (1988): 198–203.

Wise, R., U. Hadar, D. Howard, and K. Patterson. "Language Activation Studies with Positron Emission Tomography." *CIBA Foundation Symposia* 163 (1991): 218–228; discussion, 228–234.

Wittgenstein, Ludwig. *Philosophical Investigations.* Oxford: Basil Blackwell, 1986.

———. *On Certainty.* San Francisco: Arion Press, 1991.

Wolf, Alfred P. "PETT — Quantitative in vivo Measurement of Human Function and Metabolism." In *Frontiers of Analytical Techniques and Their Application: Proceedings of the Fourth Philip Morris Science Symposium, Richmond, Virginia, October 29, 1981,* Carol Greenslit Lunsford, ed., 1981a.

———. "Special Characteristics and Potential for Radiopharmaceuticals for Positron Emission Tomography." *Seminars in Nuclear Medicine* 11, no. 1 (1981b): 2–12.

Wood, William P. *Rampage.* New York: St. Martin's Press, 1985.

Wu, J. C., M. S. Buchsbaum, T. G. Hershey, et al. "PET in Generalized Anxiety Disorder." *Biological Psychiatry* 29, no. 12 (1991): 1181–1199.

Yamamoto, M., D. C. Ficke, and M. M. Ter-Pogossian. "Effect of the Software Coincidence Timing Window in Time-of-Flight Assisted Positron Emission Tomography." *IEEE Transactions on Nuclear Science* (1983) 30: 711–714.

Yamamoto, M., G. R. Hoffman, D. C. Ficke, and M. M. Ter-Pogossian. "Imaging Algorithm and Image Quality in Time-of-Flight Assisted Positron Computed Tomography: SUPER PETT I." Paper delivered at Workshop on Time-of-Flight Tomography, May 17–19, 1982, Washington University, St. Louis, Mo.

Zametkin, Alan J., Thomas E. Nordahl, Michael Gross, et al. "Cerebral Glucose Metabolism in Adults with Hyperactivity of Childhood Onset." *New England Journal of Medicine* 323, no. 20 (1990): 1361–1366.

Zimmerman, R. E. "The Developing Technology of Imaging Detectors." *Journal of Nuclear Medicine Technology* 1 (1988): 25–30.

Index of Names

General Index

Citations in italics refer to figures in the text.

accelerators. *See* cyclotrons, 37
acetylcholine, 181–182
activation. *See* brain activation
Advance Radiology (journal), 134
ADHD. *See* attention deficit hyperactivity disorder
AEC. *See* Atomic Energy Commission
Alcoholics Anonymous, 162, 205n.32
algorithms, 29, 46, 55–56, 59, 77–80, 84–88, 194. *See also* positron emission tomography experiments, algorithms in
Alzheimer's disease, 104, 129, 150, 181, 200n.6
Amgen, 183
amniocentesis, 165, 185
angiography, 23
anthropology 14, 163, 206; and ethnohistory, 31; cultural, 10; medical, 157; philosophical, 176–177, 182, 206; of science, 1, 143
antidepressant, 8, 157, 158. *See also* Prozac
anxiety, 23, 64–65, 147, 153, 206n.6
Association of Social Anthropologists of the Commonwealth, 207n.16
assumptions: as efficient, 10; about brain modules, 80–81, 83; about brain regions, 75–76; about human nature, 15, 60, 141, 144, 169, 173; in modeling,

197n.34; as necessary, 9–10; as provisional, 10; about types of persons, 22, 56, 62–63, 86–89; about types of brains, 56, 86–89. *See also* brains, types of; persons, types of; normality, derivation of
Atomic Energy Commission (AEC), 28–29
attention deficit hyperactivity disorder (ADHD), 104–105, Plate 18
authorship, 40, 57, 60, 159
autism, 104
automation, 17, 57, 87, 118, 121, 123, 170, 184; as a black box, 71
automatic computerized transverse axial (ACTA) scans, 118, 200n.1. *See* computerized tomography
autoradiography, 39, 46, 48, 91

Banister phenomenon, 34, 35
behavior: as aberrant, 202; and "abnormal brains," 126, 141, 147; as biologically controlled, 134; assumptions of in PET research, 15, 22, 59, 61, 64, 169, 175; and biochemical research, 45–46, 56; and criminality, 119, 123–124; and folk psychology, 162; and free will, 106; of neurons, 190; and PET, 26, 39; as "produced" by brains, 161; and social conditioning, 156–157

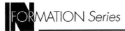FORMATION *Series*